Chinese Medical Concepts in Urban China

Martin Böke

Chinese Medical Concepts in Urban China

Change and Persistence

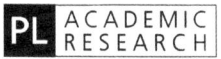

Bibliographic Information published by the Deutsche Nationalbibliothek
The Deutsche Nationalbibliothek lists this publication
in the Deutsche Nationalbibliografie; detailed bibliographic
data is available in the internet at http://dnb.d-nb.de.

Zugl.: Köln, Univ., Diss., 2013

Library of Congress Cataloging-in-Publication Data
Böke, Martin, 1980-
Chinese medical concepts in urban China : change and persistence /
Martin Böke.
pages cm
Includes bibliographical references.
Zugl.: Köln, Univ., Diss., 2013.
ISBN 978-3-631-64602-1 — ISBN 978-3-653-03864-4 (E-Book)
1. Medical care—China. 2. Medicine, Chinese. 3. Urban health—China. I. Title.
RA395.C53B65 2014
610.951—dc23
                                        2013049720

ISBN 978-3-631-64602-1 (Print)
E-ISBN 978-3-653-03864-4 (E-Book)
DOI 10.3726/978-3-653-03864-4

© Peter Lang GmbH
Internationaler Verlag der Wissenschaften
Frankfurt am Main 2014
All rights reserved.
PL Academic Research is an Imprint of Peter Lang GmbH.

Peter Lang – Frankfurt am Main · Bern · Bruxelles · New York ·
Oxford · Warszawa · Wien

All parts of this publication are protected by copyright. Any
utilisation outside the strict limits of the copyright law, without
the permission of the publisher, is forbidden and liable to
prosecution. This applies in particular to reproductions,
translations, microfilming, and storage and processing in
electronic retrieval systems.

www.peterlang.com

Table of content

I. Acknowledgements 7
II. List of Figures and Tables 9
1. Introduction 13
    Raising the Subject 14
    A Short History of Medicine in China 19
    Medical Pluralism and the Contemporary Situation of Chinese Medicine in China 29
    Excursion: Ethnology and Emotions 36

2. Research Questions and Methodology 45

3. Emotions and Health in Classical Chinese Texts 53

4. Overview of Emotions and Health in Modern Medical Textbooks 73

5. Somatization – 'Eastern Culture-bound Syndrome' or 'Western Culture-bound Perspective'? 81

6. Empirical Results 87
    Beijing Inhabitant's Familiarity with Chinese Medical Concepts and the Evaluation of Chinese Medicine 122
    The Pathological Potential of Emotions 124
    Group-specific perception of illnesses caused by emotions 127
    Utilization of Chinese medicine 130
    The Experts' Interviews 132

7. Specific Answering Patterns 149
    Age-specific Peculiarities: Changing Habitus and Different Modes of Power 149

Education-specific Peculiarities: Stress, Depression and the Chinese
Education System 163
Gender-specific Peculiarities: 'Superior Births' and
'Superior Mothers' 168

8. Conclusion: Chinese Medicine Between Change and Persistence 175

9. Appendices 183
Appendix 1: Questionnaire 183
Appendix 2: Statistical Data of the Survey 187
Appendix 3: Information on Medical Experts and
Medical Institutions 188

10. References 191

I. Acknowledgements

I gratefully acknowledge the support and help of many individuals and several institutions who supported me on various occasions during the last years. I am indebted to their help, criticism and encouragement.
    First of all, I am indebted to my PhD-thesis supervisor Prof. Dr. Michael J. Casimir (this book is based on my PhD-thesis, University of Cologne 2013). The German term "Doktorvater" is a nice description, for it reveals a deeper insight in how the relationship between teacher and student can be shaped ideally. I am happy to have found a teacher who supported me throughout my study in waking my curiosity in Cultural Anthropology and especially in Medical Anthropology, but who also became a good friend and advisor. He not only was a dedicated teacher to me, but he is also constantly a critical and inspiring discussion partner.
    Additionally, my thanks go to my second supervisor, Prof. Dr. Michael Bollig, who also encouraged me in my endeavours, provided me with useful contacts and established far-reaching academic relationships.
    Furthermore I would like to thank the staff of the Institute of Cultural and Social Anthropology of the University of Cologne with its director, Prof. Dr. Martin Rössler. They supported me in my scholarly interest through many years.
    I am also indebted to the Chinese Academy of Social Sciences, to the Beijing Minzu University (北京中央民族大学) and its Institute of Ethnology and Anthropology, namely to Prof. Dr. Zhang Jijiao, Prof. Du Fachun and especially to Prof. Zhang Xiaomin. They were a great and attentive help during my field visits in Beijing, inspiring conversation partners and hospitable hosts. Additionally, I like to thank cordially Dr. Wang Yuan, Dr. Wang Xiuxiao and Dr. Sun Xiaoshu, who helped me carrying out my research, facilitated helpful contacts and furthermore helped me to avoid loneliness in my field site. They were not only reliable and indispensable research assistants and inspiring colleagues, but also warm-hearted friends.
    The realization of this whole project would have been impossible without the support of the a.r.t.e.s. Forschungsschule, the graduate school of the University of Cologne. A.r.t.e.s. as an institution supported me financially with a scholarship, but furthermore, the people building up a.r.t.e.s. helped me developing my ideas, constantly reviewed my project and enlarged my scholarly focus. Especially I would like to thank the spokesperson of a.r.t.e.s., Prof. Dr. Dr. h.c. Andreas Speer, for his constant interest and encouragement and his ability to

create a good and expedient institution with a fruitful working atmosphere. Furthermore, I would like to thank the members of the a.r.t.e.s. Class 5, who made useful suggestions on my project.

Equally impossible would the project have been without the obliging and helpful manner of the inhabitants of Beijing. This is true for the nameless, common people on the streets, who, with no word of irritation, haste or rejection, answered my questions patiently, tried to help me when I was struggling with my Chinese, or just were nice and friendly interviewees. Furthermore, this is true for the staff of the medical institutions I visited and which have to stay anonymous in this book on their own accord. They spent their time to answer my questions patiently and to satisfy my curiosity, showed me their working places and explained their attitudes and opinion openly and without hesitation. I am indebted to all of my informants: the collected data, and consequently the backbone of this book, all stems from their patience and helpfulness.

Truly I am indebted to my family. My parents constantly supported me, not only financially on more than one occasion, but also ideationally. I owe to my brother, Dr. Simon Boeke, several interesting debates about biomedical attitudes and practices, and additionally he helped me to understand complicated biomedical issues.

And I would like to thank my Julia for her constant support, for being my source of happiness and contentedness, and for catching me up several times when I was about to struggle.

Cologne, August 2013

Martin Boeke

II. List of Figures, Tables and Abbrevations

Figures

Fig. 1: The yin yang-Symbol 22
Fig. 2: Political slogans concerning the relationship between Chinese
and Western medicine 32
Fig. 3: Map of the city centre of Beijing with the 4th ring road 47
Fig. 4: Distribution of gender in age groups among survey participants 50
Fig. 5: Pathogenesis of Heart Disease 77
Fig. 6: Pathogenesis of Liver Disease 78
Fig. 7: Aetiology of Depression 79
Fig. 8: Investigation areas 89
Fig. 9: Distribution of gender in age groups among survey participants 90
Fig. 10: Distribution of survey participants according to city districts 91
Fig. 11: Can emotions induce illnesses? 92
Fig. 12: Most frequently mentioned illness terms 93
Fig. 13a: Illnesses caused by emotions: age-specific answering patterns 95
Fig. 13b: Illnesses caused by emotions: age-specific answering patterns 96
Fig. 14: Organs perceived as being potentially influenced by emotions 97
Fig. 15: Knowledge and evaluation of the book 'Huangdi neijing' 100
Fig. 16: Self-reported knowledge of certain Chinese medical concepts 101
Fig. 17: Self-reported lack of knowledge of Chinese medical concepts
according to education 102
Fig. 18: Numbers of emotions named as belonging to the 'Seven Emotions'.. 103
Fig. 19: Self-reported knowledge of 'psychotherapy'
(jingshen liaofa 精神疗法) according to age groups 106
Fig. 20: Perceived meaning of the term 'psychotherapy'
(jingshen liaofa 精神疗法) according to age groups 107
Fig. 21: Sources of medical knowledge 108
Fig. 22: Perceived availability of different medical systems in Beijing 110
Fig. 23: Reported consultation of different medical systems in the last year .. 111
Fig. 24: Reported consultation of different medical systems
in the last year by men 112
Fig. 25: Reported consultations of different medical systems
in the last year by women 113
Fig. 26: Attitudes on Chinese medicine: distribution of sum-scores 116
Fig. 27: Attitudes on Chinese medicine: distribution of sum-scores

according to age 117
Fig. 28: Attitudes on Chinese medicine: distribution of sum-scores
according to gender 118
Fig. 29: Attitudes on pathological potential of emotions: distribution
of sum-scores.. 120
Fig. 30: Attitudes on pathological potential of emotions: distribution of
sum-scores according to educational background 121
Fig. 31: Young Red Guards on a cover of a 1971 schoolbook 129
Fig. 32: Billboards advertising women's hospitals in Beijing 132
Fig. 33: Picture of a so called 'struggle session' (1967, Shenyang)................. 159
Fig. 34: The 'Haidian district healthcare clinic for mothers and infants" haidianqu fuyou boajian yuan 海淀区妇幼保健院) 171

Tables:

Table 1: The 'Five Phases' 24
Table 2: The Zangfu Organs 26
Table 3: Question categories and exemplarily questions asked during
experts' interviews 134

Abbreviations:

CCP	Chinese Communist Party
CM	Chinese Medicine
GMD	Guomindang
HDNJ	Huangdi Neijing
NJ	Nanjing
TCM	Traditional Chinese Medicine

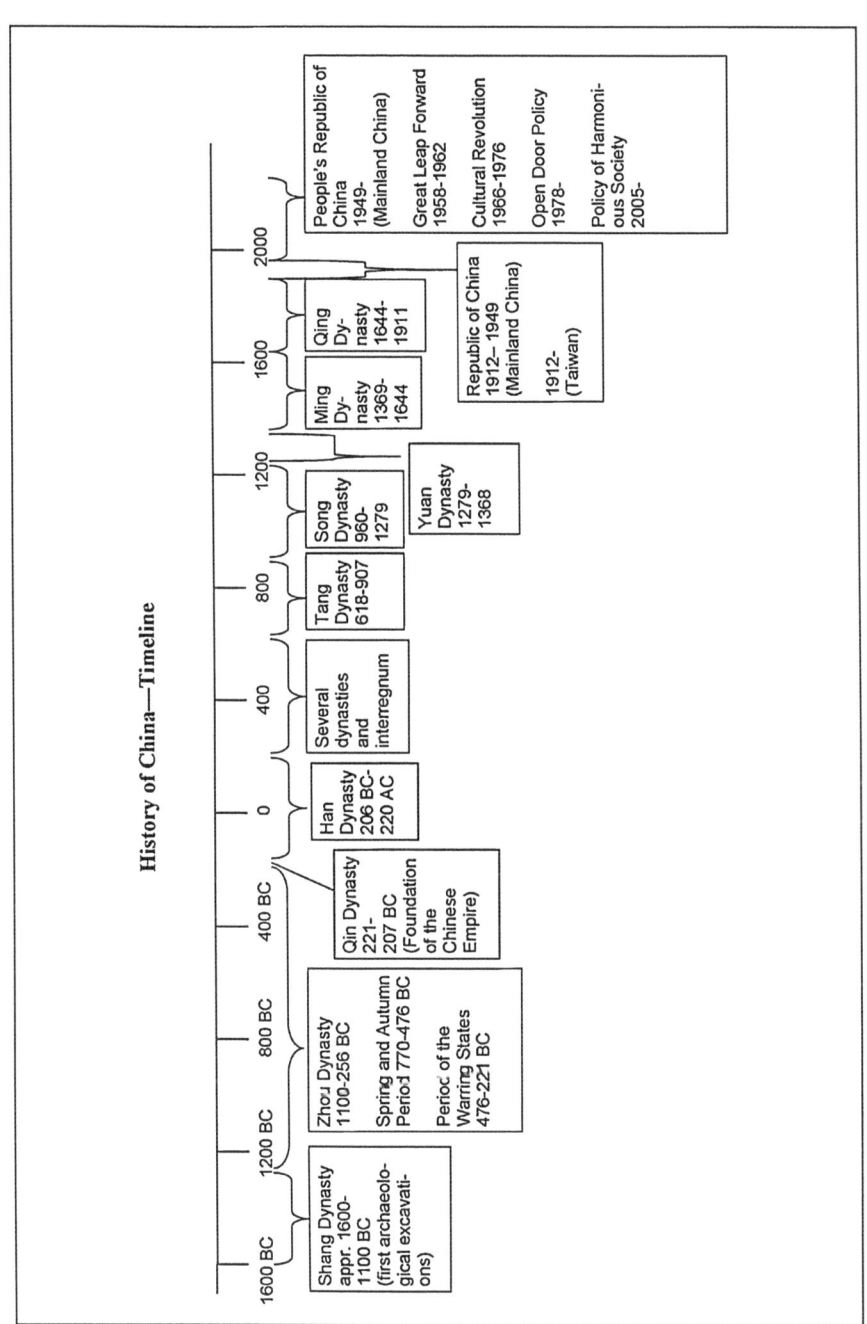

1. Introduction

Popular assertions outbid each other with the history, tradition and founding period of Chinese medicine, proclaiming a tradition of 2000 years[1], of 4000 years[2], or of even more than 5000 years[3]. Even while acknowledging a long history and tradition, is this really important for today's China? Has Chinese medicine relevance for modern, cosmopolitan urban Chinese today? Do these people know something about its disease concepts or pathogenic mechanisms of action? Do they regard these theories and categories of illnesses as relevant? And, as China's political system changed several times dramatically during the last century, do these changes influence the people's estimation of illnesses? These are some questions which I would like to elucidate in this thesis.

I mainly focus on emotions and their relevance in Chinese medicine. Emotions build one disease category in Chinese medicine, the 'Seven Emotions'. This feature is commonly praised in popular discourse as *'ganzheitlich'* or holistic. Because of this popularity, and because of my interest in human emotionality, I specialized on this feature of Chinese medicine for wider parts of this book.

The book is structured as follows: after this preface, I give an introduction encompassing three subchapters. First, I raise the subject and provide information about the field site. Second, I outline the history of Chinese medicine and explain main theories and concepts. Lastly, I present an overview of main assumptions of ethnological research on human emotions. The second chapter clarifies the research questions and the methodology. In the third chapter, I present an overview on the connections between emotions and illnesses in classical Chinese texts, summarizing first philosophical texts, divided into Confucian, Daoist and others, and second resuming classical medical texts on this topic, starting with very important and influential texts like the *huangdi neijing*. Afterwards, in the fourth chapter, I outline the connections between emotions and illnesses in selected modern textbooks on Chinese medicine, followed by a chapter discussing the concept of 'somatization'. In the sixth chapter I present

---

1   en.wikipedia.org: http://en.wikipedia.org/wiki/Traditional_Chinese_medicine ; last access 20.06.2012.
2   www.shen-nong.com: http://www.shen-nong.com/eng/history/chronology.html#origin ; last access 20.06.2012.
3   www.purifymind.com: http://www.purifymind.com/HistoryMed.htm ; last access 20.06.2012.

the empirical results, both of my survey and of my expert interviews, and discussing these results in broader context. Subsequently I append the seventh chapter analysing group specific answering-patterns and –behaviour, namely, age-specific, education-specific, and gender-specific peculiarities. I argue that age-specific differences in the perception of depression are related to the experience of different modes of power. Education-specific stress and pressure is connected to the perception of education as capital. The gender-specific utilization of Western medicine has to be analysed considering the discourses on superior births and superior mothers. In my concluding eighth chapter, I summarize the main observations.

The following introduction is tripartite: First, I raise the subject, give an explanation as to why I chose Chinese medicine and provide initial information about the situation in the field; secondly, I give an outline of Chinese medicine, the main concepts, the history and also the recent situation of medical pluralism in China; finally, I summarise the main assumptions of ethnological research on human emotions by introducing emotions both as "complex reactions in the struggle of survival" (Plutchik 1982: 551) and as "embodied thought" (Rosaldo 1984: 143).

By doing so, I will lay the foundation for the upcoming effectuations and intend to facilitate the comprehensibility. Some aspects will be redundant, for which I hope their repetition is both justifiable and excusable.

Raising the Subject

Medical Anthropology, earlier termed Ethnomedicine, is a sub-discipline of Cultural Anthropology and deals specifically with the whole complex of human existence within the context of illness and health. Once defined as

> [Ethnomedicine is] the study of how members of different cultures think about disease and organize themselves toward medical treatment and the social organization of treatment itself (Fabrega 1975: 969),

the broader context of human life and especially the historical, sociological, economical, and political implications of disease and healing have been investigated more and more in the last decades (Fabrega 1990a: 129 f.). Starting with Arthur Kleinman's investigations in the early 1970s, 'modern' Medical Anthropology tried to overcome the long lasting prejudices of scientific Western medicine versus superstitious 'primitive' medicine or, less offensive but nevertheless discriminating, between "personalistic" and "naturalistic" medicine (Kleinman 1978a: 661-662). Within the complex construct of "health, illness and healing in society as a cultural system" (Kleinman 1978b: 85), the investigation of this system has much more to offer than just an interaction between healer and patient. There is a process to be analyzed which connects the concepts of diseases and its ideas about the origin of illnesses to the personal experience of being ill, to a certain pattern of behaviour, to decision-making processes, to the actual therapeutic intervention and to the retrospective analysis of the illness episode (ibid. 86). In this study I shall investigate these manifold interconnections and try to link certain perceptions of illness origins and certain decisions for health treatment and therapeutic interventions to historical, political and economical factors. In Singer's sense that "disease [...] must be understood as the product of historically located socio-political processes" (Singer & Baer 1995: 90), I proceed by saying that disease concepts must be understood also as a product of historically located socio-political processes. To avoid the cliché of a static medical system resting on the two columns of Western medicine and traditional medicine, I shall follow Margaret Lock's interjection demanding "multifocality" (Lock 2007: 270). Hence, by providing a structured survey, I will analyze the illness concepts of common urban people in China's capital Beijing, as diverse as these people may be. Additionnaly, I will outline the views of professionals, medical staff as well as administrative. Furthermore, I will evaluate the many individual voices which came up during informal interviews with common people on the streets. Consequently, this study is not only "multifocal" but also 'multiphonic'.

The Western discussion concerning so called 'alternative' medical systems and the search unorthodox cures of '*Schulmedizin*' (mainstream Western medicine or biomedicine) has noticeably picked up pace in the last two decades. The choice of medical alternatives in German cities is enormous; ranging from small offices of self-trained alternative healers to officially labelled '*Heilpraktiker*' (alternative practitioner) and culminates in doctors who not only received a license ('*Approbation*') to practice biomedicine, but also engaged in extensive studies of written systems like the Indian Ayurvedic System or the system of

Traditional Chinese Medicine[4]. As for the last mentioned system, there are a multitudinous number of publications in Western languages, especially in German. One may find that the vast majority of these publications focus not so much on the community of social scientists but on the broader public which is quite understandable. The 'alternative' medicines are a broad market and generate values of more than 9 billion Euros a year in Germany (Spielberg 2007: 3148). Even German health insurance companies, normally very adverse to 'alternative' curing methods, reimburse some specific 'alternative' medical treatments rooted in Chinese medical thought.[5] To demonstrate the intensive contact with, at least a partial representative of, Chinese medicine, one can see that the density of acupuncturists in Germany (2000 inhabitants per acupuncturist) is even higher than in mainland China (4000 inhabitants per acupuncturist).[6] Interestingly enough, acupuncture and the closely related technique of moxibustion seems to be a *pars pro toto* for Chinese medicine in the West ever since: Even the earliest Western reports on Chinese medical practices, for example the letters written by the German Jesuit missionary Johannes Schreck (1576-1630) or the letters of the physician Andreas Cleyer (1615-1690) addressed to the *Collegium Naturae Curiosum* in Schweinfurt, focused mainly on these techniques (Michel 1993: 215-216; 2005: 71-72). Recently the UNESCO labelled the techniques of acupuncture and moxibustion as "Intangible Cultural Heritages of Humanity".[7] To label a medical practice as "intangible culture" is at least discussible. But by doing so, the UNESCO cemented the notion of Chinese medicine as mainly consisting of this technique and, to a certain extent, neglects the possibility and opportunity for change.

---

4   With the term "Traditional Chinese Medicine" (TCM) I label a specific part of the broader system "Chinese medicine" (CM). For the clarification of these two terms, see subchapter 1.2.2.
5   Since April 16th 2006 reimbursement by treating chronic knee-pain, back-pain and headache with acupuncture will be provided (http://www.krankenkassen.de/gesetzliche-krankenkassen/leistungen-gesetzliche-krankenkassen/gesetzlich-vorgeschriebene-leistungen/neue-leistungen/akupunktur-kassenleistung/) (latest access 09.05.2011).
6   Press release from 02.01.2011 by the „Deutsches Institut für Traditionelle Chinesische Medizin e.V. (DITCM)" (http://www.tcm.de/html/aktuell__unesco-akupunktur.html) (latest access 09.05.2011).
7   UNESCO Homepage (http://www.unesco.org/culture/ich/index.php?RL=00425) (latest access 09.05.2011).

Why China?

Despite all the interest in and sometimes even euphoria over 'alternative' medical practices, there is one limitation for the cultural anthropologist: China has not been on the agenda for most Western anthropologists and Chinese medicine and its role in modern China is discussed in only two handfuls of ethnographies; for example, the books by Judith Farquhar (1994a), Thomas Ots (1999), Elisabeth Hsu (1999), Volker Scheid (2002) or Zhang Yanhua (2007a); although since Charles Leslie (1976) medical anthropologists also focussed on Nonwestern canonized medical systems. The few existing ethnographies have in common that they mainly deal with the sphere of medical 'experts'. Farquhar (1994a), for example, describes how knowledge is being passed on in the context of a big clinic as well as in the more personal relationship between master and disciple. Ots (1999) outlines the principles of Chinese medicine and shows the clinical reality by giving some case studies whereas Scheid (2002) tries to explain why for practitioners of Chinese medicine, there is no conflict between being 'traditional' and being 'modern'. All these great ethnographies left one aspect widely un-noted, and therefore provide an opportunity for more research centred upon analyzing the knowledge and attitudes of lay-persons and gathering information about their usage and contextualisation of indigenous illness concepts.

As Chinese medicine is such a popular topic in Germany right now, I wondered about the situation in China itself. The country is developing swiftly, adapting Western techniques and knowledge as well as attitudes and lifestyles in such a rapid way while combining them with Chinese legacies; thereby giving the well networked and highly skilled urban inhabitants the opportunity – at least in a certain, governmentally approved framework – to make choices and to behave individually, maybe for the first time in Chinese history (c.f. Yan 2009). What about the medical system? Is a system that claims a history of more than 2000 years still attractive and relevant to young urban professionals, colloquially termed, 'Yuppies' (*yapi* 雅皮), which are focused on status and consumption?[8]

---

8   Yan (2000: 169) illustrates vividly the changed patterns of consumption of Chinese urban population. The "three big items" (san da jian 三大件) which were most desirable in the 1960s and 1970s were wristwatches, bicycles and sewing machines. In the 1980s, these items were color TVs, refrigerators and washing machines, whereas these were replaced by telephones, air conditioners and VCRs in the early 1990s. In the late 1990s

Or instead, do only older people know the mysterious remedies and old secrets of Chinese medicine? Are they sceptical of Western medicine and do they lament the 'good old times' of Chinese medicine?

The Situation in the Field

Initially, during the initial planning of the research project, I thought of doing a classical ethnological rural-urban comparison, because I estimated (and I still do) that the differences between the situation in rural and urban China must also be reflected in the attitudes and assessments of Chinese medical concepts and that there are some important and relevant distinctions in the way people make sense of Chinese medical concepts and make use of Chinese medicine. For the sake of time and space, I narrowed it down to the observation of the urban society. This decision allowed for an intimate investigation of the urban population's attitude and usage of Chinese medicine; focusing on rural attitudes and usages would have detracted from the comparability to other urban studies, which I try to stress in my analysis. I think, conducting fieldwork in a rural area and repeating my questions there would be a good and worthwhile supplemental venture; a rural-urban comparison would obtain interesting results, but it would shift the study in a different direction away from an urban foucs which I provide in this study.

So I decided to do the fieldwork in urban China, but I was not quite sure which city I should select. I finally chose Beijing for several reasons. First of all, it is the capital and therefore a kind of prototype for Chinese cities. Although some Chinese city dwellers wondered about this choice, as they considered Beijing backward, provincial and boring and recommended cities like Shanghai to be the better, more modern and more urban spot, I chose Beijing. At least since the run-up to the Olympic Games in 2008, the city developed the awareness of not only of being the head of Chinese bureaucracy, but also modern and internationally relevant. Beside this, Beijing "along with the Great Wall is the dominant symbol of 5,000 years of Chinese history and tradition" (de Kloet 2002: 99). Beijing proved to be the ideal choice because of its relevance in economical and political power, and because of its efforts to combine the emerging image of a modern metropolis and the tradition of being the Chinese capital, although with

---

and in the beginning 2000s, the new three big items are apartments, private cars and modern cell phones.

discontinuities, for almost 800 years. It hosts the University for Chinese Medicine (*Beijing Zhongyiyao Daxue*北京中医药大学) as well as other important institutions, both academic and government, concerning health and medicine. And also some more pragmatic reasons, which every ethnologist doubtlessly has, but hesitantly talks about, were decisive. I knew the city quite well due to previous travels, and also the local dialect which is close to 'mandarin' or standard Chinese was an important factor. For example, conversation with a dialect speaker from southern China would have complicated my research demonstrably.[9]

I chose to stay in the north-western part of Beijing, close to the Renmin University (*Renmin Daxue* 人民大学) and to the Central University for Nationalities (*Zhongyang Minzu Daxue*中央民族大学) where I had my main contacts and connections. In the second chapter, I will expound upon the research sites. Interviews took place in different locations, but all inside the 4th ring road of Beijing in the city centre and the nearest suburbs.

A Short History of Medicine in China

As already mentioned, the ethnological discussion about indigenous medical concepts in China, at least in Germany, has not been very polyphonic in the last few decades and also lacks a recent history (c.f. Unschuld 1991: 63-64) and so a brief description of Chinese medical thought is needed to provide a backdrop. In modern China, not only Chinese medicine but also Western medicine is known and 'theoretically' available; summarizing the history of medicine in China since the establishment of the first educational institution for Western medicine in China at the very beginning of the 20th century until present is needed.

Discoveries from different archaeological excavations can verify that already during *Shang Dynasty* (*shang chao* 商朝 ; approx. 16. - 11.cent. B.C.), so called "oracle medicine" was popular and common in parts today called China. Animal bones and tortoise shells were scratched[10] and exposed to fire. By interpreting the fracture lines, the shaman could give advices to the person seeking help

---

9   Chinese dialects are very diverging and in the worst case incompatible to standard Chinese.
10 From these scratched symbols the first Chinese characters derived.

(Jewell 1990: 221). There was not yet any kind of specialization for medical experts because predictions of misfortune of all kinds, from bad harvest to natural disaster and disease as well as advice on how to deal with these misfortunes were commonly offered by the same oracle. The existence of solely medical experts is not verified for this period (Ots 1999: 41), although from the findings of bronze knifes and needles, experts draw the conclusion that surgery must have not been uncommon during these times (Ho & Lisowski 1993: 8). Beside the excavation findings, there is other evidence for the roots of Chinese medicine in oracle séances. An old version of the character for medicine (*yi*) is written with the elements 'arrow and quiver' (*yi*医), 'bamboo lance' (*shu* 殳) and 'shaman' (*wu* 巫) (Unschuld 2006: 45). The weapons symbolize the fight of the shaman against the evil powers that sap the patient's energy and cause the disease. Around the 3rd century B.C., shamans lost their important and powerful social position.[11] Simultaneously, a new medical branch was developing and gained importance; medical drug therapy. As most of these drugs were mixed with alcoholic liquids, the character for 'alcohol' (*jiu* 酒) replaced the character for 'shaman' around the 3rd century B.C. and constitutes with the two other elements, 'arrow and quiver' (*yi* 医) and 'bamboo lance' (*shu*殳), the character for medicine *yi* 醫 until today (Unschuld 2006: 46).[12]

The roots of medicine in China are explored in the classic 'Handbook of the Yellow Emperor on Inner Medicine' (*Huangdi neijing* 皇帝內經 (HDNJ)). This book is attributed to the mythological 'Yellow Emperor', a cultural hero which is said to have lived more than 4500 years ago and founded the Chinese culture. Today, the HDNJ is dated to the 3rd or 2nd century B.C. It is a compilation of different older scriptures by unknown authors and tries to combine and edit the transmission of medical knowledge (Hsu 2005: 12). Through conducting numerous interviews and observations, it has been found to still be relevant today as a standard reference for Chinese medical experts and seen as a core element of Chinese medicine.

The following pages outline a brief review of main concepts in Chinese medicine, starting with the general evaluation of harmony. Subsequently, the

---

11 See Wang 2005. The author shows that the character for 'defamation' (wu 诬) is derived from 'shaman' and 'talking' so that symbolically the words of the shaman became lies and deception.

12 On mainland China there has been a reform and simplification of the characters starting in 1956, so that the character yi now is only written with the element 'arrow and quiver' 医. In Hong Kong and Taiwan these simplified characters are not used, so there the character yi still consists of the three mentioned elements, although the part for "alcohol" lost the three dots on the left side, or the 'three dots of water' (san dian shui三点水)

concepts of *qi* and *yin* and *yang* are outlined, followed by an explanation of the system of 'Five Phases'. Thereupon succeeds the description of anatomic and pathologic concepts and an overview of aspects of demonic medicine.

The Concept of Harmony

The two crucial philosophical schools which shaped Chinese society for centuries and to this day still have great influence, Daoism and Confucianism, broke new ground during the highly unstable periods of the 'Spring and Autumn Period' (*chunqiu shidai*春秋时代 , 722-482 B.C.) and the 'Warring States Period' (*zhanguo shidai* 战国时代 , 481-221 B.C.), the foundational periods for Chinese philosophy.[13] The opinions and ideas of these two schools influenced the authors of the HDNJ demonstrably and have one thing in common: they both strive for harmony, albeit in different ways. Daoism tries to achieve 'the way' (*dao* 道) to harmony through the technique of 'acting through non-acting' (*wu wei* 無爲 / 无为), whereas Confucianism is far away from non-acting but promotes the strict observation of rules and moral standards as 'virtue' (*de* 德) or 'filial piety' (*xiao* 孝).[14] For example, the ancient classics 'Book of Rites' (*Liji* 禮記)[15] and '*Xunzi*' (荀子)[16] both state that violation of the rules leads to disorder: on the macroscopic level, the disorder of state and society; on microscopic level, personal illness and suffering. However, achieving harmony through obeying the rules leads to a prosperous and healthy state as well as to healthy individuals (Böke 2008: 16).[17]

---

13   While talking of Chinese philosophy, these two periods are sometimes summarized under the name 'Hundred Schools of Thought' (Zhuzi Baijia 諸子百家).
14   For further information about Chinese philosophy see for example Fung 1983, Ivanhoe & van Norden 2001, Liu 2006. For contemporary Chinese philosophy see Cheng & Bunnin 2002.
15   One of the five classics of the Confucian canon.
16   A collection of writings by the author of the same name, Confucian philosopher (appr. 312-230 B.C.).
17   For detailed information and discussion about the ancient texts see chapter 3.

The Concepts of qi 氣, yin 陰 and yang 陽

From my point of view, a translation of these concepts in any Western language is impossible because of the implications of these concepts. As Ots puts it, *qi* has a tangible and material as well as an energetic and functional element (Ots 1999: 59). These two components are visible in the character 氣 which consists of the two parts: 'air' or 'vapour' (*qi* 气) and 'rice' (*mi* 米). By combining the two preconditions of live, air and sustenance, one can already estimate the importance of *qi* in Chinese medical thoughts. As *qi* has a supplying function, every congestion and blockade of it inevitably leads to illness. It is omni-present and nothing in the world can exist without it.[18] Depending on the lifecycle, there is a different *qi* status in a person. Additionally, different organs have specific states of *qi* which should be maintained in order to preserve health. It was suggested by the informants that different *qi* states are the answer to certain illnesses.

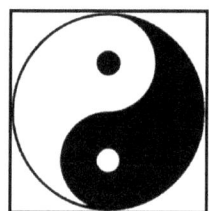

Fig. 1: The yin yang-Symbol

Originally the terms *yin* and *yang* indicated the shadowed (*yin*) and the sunny (*yang*) side of a hill. This meaning can still be reconstructed by looking at the characters; *yin* 陰 on the one hand includes the element for 'cloud' (*yun* 云) while *yang* 陽, on the other hand, includes the element 'sun' (*ri* 日). However, for the early philosophers, this concrete meaning dwindled away towards a more general dichotomy; for example, the opposition of dark and light, or female and male. One medical implication is that *yin* has a more conserving role whereas

---

18   See also Hsu 2003 and 1999. Her research shows that qi gained increased significance during the totalitarian sovereignty of the Western Han Dynasty (3rd cent. A.C.): "Als universales Medium, das alles durchdringt, das dialektisch Kultur und Natur miteinander verbindet, das in den fernsten Punkt des Kaiserreiches gelangen wie auch in den innersten Teil des menschlichen Körpers eindringen kann, und das sich auch lokal verändern kann und dem Örtlichen angleicht, war qi als Konzept Bestandteil einer Herrschaft, die nach universaler Autorität trachtete." (Hsu 2003: 186).

yang is a more dynamic factor (Ots 1999: 45). As visible in the well know symbol (Fig. 1), *yin* incorporates a small dose of *yang* and vice versa.[19] *Yin* and *yang* are also required to be in a harmonious condition. As the 'Book of Changes' (*Yijing* 易經)[20] puts it: "一 陰 一 陽 之 謂 道" – "One *yin* and one *yang* leads to *dao*" (*Yijing*, *Xi Ci* 1, 5; also see Böke 2008: 18).

The 'Five Phases' (*wuxing* 五行)

In older publications, this concept is frequently translated as 'Five Elements'; this is certainly an oversimplification.[21] Actually, this concept's character is a very dynamic one as an everlasting circulation and mutual connections and influences are postulated. The five basic elements of 'wood' (*mu*木), 'fire' (*huo*火), 'earth' (*tu*土), 'metal' (*jin*金) and 'water' (*shui*水) are connected on a macroscopic level (seasons, cardinal directions, climate, colour etc.) and on a microscopic level (organs, emotions, orifices, tissues etc.), as shown in Table 1.

---

19   This symbol (Taijitu 太極圖 / 太极图) is not proved in China before the 11th century A.C. and is regularly used only since the Ming Dynastie (1368-1644) (see Robinet 2008).
20   (One of) the oldest Chinese classics, written in the mid 4th century B.C.
21   The meanings of the characters are 'five' (五) and 'walking' or 'moving' (行).

Table 1: The 'Five Phases' (Kaptchuk 2000: 439).

	Wood (*mu* 木)	Fire (*huo* 火)	Earth (*tu* 土)	Metal (*jin* 金)	Water (*shui* 水)
season	Spring	Summer	"Indian summer"	Autumn	Winter
direction	East	South	Centre	West	North
climate	Windy	Hot	Damp	Dry	Cold
colour	Green	Red	Yellow	White	Black
yin-organ	Liver	Heart	Spleen	Lungs	Kidney
yang-organ	Gall Bladder	Small Intestine	Stomach	Large Intestine	Bladder
emotion	Anger	Elation	Pensiveness	Grief	Fear
orifice	Eyes	Tongue	Mouth	Nose	Ears
tissue	Tendons	Blood vessels	Flesh	Skin	Bones

The three cycles of emergence, overcoming and overpowering are induced by the two fundamental principles of 'mutual emergence' (*xiangsheng* 相生) and 'mutual conquest' (*xiangke* 相克) (Ho & Lisowski 1993: 16). The connections and correspondence of the different aspects of one phase are more or less based empirically. For example, the spring lets the plants turn green and trees grow, while in certain parts of China there is wind from the eastern direction. On the microscopic level, we can state that the liver and gall bladder build a functional unit. Liver diseases can be revealed in the eyes. When people are angry, the tendons in the neck and in the extremities are strained. The connection between anger and the liver can be observed in many cultures; it is a mystery why, of all things, the liver is connected to this emotion (because normally humans cannot 'feel' the liver, as they would, for example, a heartbeat, breathing or a movement of the bowels etc.). In the further chapters, I outline that this linkage of the liver and anger plays an important role in different contexts. My empirical results also show that the connection between the liver and emotions (in most cases anger) is still assumed by many Chinese urban citizens. Regarding the link of macroscopic and microscopic level of this specific phase (see Table 1, phase 'wood'), Ots speculates that it derives from the colloquial term 'liver wind' (*ganfeng* 肝风). 'Wind' is synonymous with certain symptoms characterized as ascending such as a headache or vertigo. These symptoms are linked to anger, which itself is characterized as suddenly appearing and frequently changing directions much like all aspects of the wind. He sees the linkage between the two levels established through the relation between wind and anger (Ots 1999: 50).

Anatomical and Pathological Concepts: 'Storage and Palace Organs' *zangfu* (脏腑 /臟 腑), 'Six Evils' (*liu xie* 六邪) and 'Seven Emotions' (*qi qing* 七情)

As demonstrated in the analysis of the ancient texts (chapter 3), there is a strong tendency to draw an analogy between the macroscopic and the microscopic as well as between the state and the body in classical Chinese thought. Just as the feudal states of ancient China consisted of palaces and storage depots, the human body is divided into 'palace-organs' (*fu* 腑) and 'storage-organs' (*zang* 脏) which are connected through a network of channels and vessels. The HDNJ also mentions this interdependence:

> The heart is the Prince of the body, the seat of the vital spirit. The lungs are the ministers who regulate one's actions. The gall bladder is the central office, courage dwells in it. The pericardium is the ambassador who brings joy and happiness. The spleen and stomach are the granaries, the five tastes emanate from them. The large intestine is the organ of communication where matters are undergoing changes. The small intestine is the receiving organ, the place of digestion. Skill proceeds from the kidney, the seat of vigour and strength. [...]" (*Huangdi neijing*, in: Jewell 1990: 232).

The storage-organs, which are related to *yin*, include the heart, lungs, spleen, liver and kidneys. Unschuld counts the pericardium as a sixth *zang*-organ (1985: 77), but Kaptchuk argues that the pericardium is not considered a *zang*-organ in the HDNJ but later in the 'Classic of Difficult Questions[22] (*Nanjing* 難經) and is not distinguished from the heart in general theory (Kaptchuk 2000: 90 & 99).

---

22 The Nanjing was written in the late Han-Dynasty, probably in the 2nd or early 3rd century A.C.

The palace-organs, related to *yang*, incorporate the gall bladder, stomach, small intestine, large intestine, bladder and the *san jiao* (三焦)[23]. Xie (2003: 41) suggests 'triple energizer' as a proper translation while others such as Jewell (1990: 231) translate it as 'triple burner'.

Table 2: The *zangfu* Organs.

Storage organs *zang*脏	Liver *gan* 肝	Heart *xin* 心	Spleen *pi* 脾	Lungs *fei* 肺	Kidneys *shen* 肾	Pericardium *xinbao* 心包
Palace organs *fu*腑	Gall Bladder *dan* 胆	Small intestine *xiaochang* 小肠	Stomach *wei* 胃	Large intestine *dachang* 大肠	Bladder *Pangguang* 膀胱	*san jiao* 三焦

While looking at the organ names, one has to keep in mind that these organs in Chinese medicine and biomedicine mean different things. The correct biomedical Chinese term for the heart, for example, is *xin* (心). In Chinese medicine, this biomedical meaning is extended and the organ *xin* 心 is not only the specific organ of the muscle and flesh, but also a 'functional circle' ("Funktionskreis", Ots 1999: 56). It includes the connections to corresponding functional circles and is seen as a part of a system, not only as a single organ.

For Chinese aetiology, the ultimate cause of illness is a disharmony of *yin* and *yang* or a blockade of *qi*. This disharmony and blockade can be caused by different factors; for example bad or inappropriate food or environmental influences. Chinese medicine differentiates between three categories of proximate causes of illness; namely the 'outer causes' (*wai yin* 外淫), the 'inner causes' (*nei yin* 内淫) and the causes which are neither outer nor inner. The outer causes

---

23 As the san jiao describes a part of the upper torso which is supposed to be responsible for metabolic processes, from my point of view there is no fitting translation and so I will leave this body part un-translated.

are called the 'Six Evils' (*liu xie*六邪) and involve the climatic phenomena 'wind' (*feng* 风), 'cold' (*han* 寒), 'fire' (*huo*火), 'dampness' (*shi* 湿), 'dryness' (*zao* 燥) and 'summer heat' (*shu* 暑). As Kaptchuk states, these Six Evils have

> the name of an atmospheric condition that is considered to be out of control, [and it] is a metaphoric representation of 'bad weather' that persists in the human terrain. The disharmonious climate has the sense that the yin-yang balance has been disrupted and distorted (Kaptchuk 2000: 146).

The inner causes are called the 'Seven Emotions' (*qi qing* 七情). In contemporary Chinese medicine, they consist of 'happiness' (*xi* 喜), 'anger' (*nu* 怒), 'worry' (*you* 忧), 'thinking' (*si* 思), 'sadness' (*bei* 悲), 'fear' (*kong* 恐) and 'fright' (*jing* 惊). Chapter 3 will contain a broader and more detailed discussion about the philosophical implications and the different composition of the Seven Emotions depending on philosophical background. For this introduction, it is enough to delineate that these emotions are connected to certain organs (see Table 1). Emotions are recognized as an integral part of human beings, but they are considered as dangerous when they are either in excess or insufficient. They can influence the corresponding organs, creating a disharmonious state, and cause imbalance and illness. 'Somatic' disorders can cause emotional instability, too (Kaptchuk 2000: 158); this medical implication of emotional experience and the deep connection between emotions and body parts is also visible in common Chinese phrases and 'proverbs' (*chengyu*成语). Happiness, for example, is expressed as having an 'open heart' (*kaixin* 开心). Wierzbicka (1999: 301) identifies more expressions like 'cutting the heart with a knife' (*xin ru dao ge* 心如刀割) meaning sadness or 'breaking the five organs' (*wu zang ju lie* 五脏决裂) meaning anger. Although these metaphorical utilizations are common in other languages, for example 'breaking one's heart' in English or '*an die Nieren gehen*' (literally: 'something affects my kidneys', meaning 'to be shocked by something') in German, these expressions are not a "philosophical-medical heritage as they are China" (Pritzker 2003: 20).

Demonic Medicine

As already stated in the etymology of the character for 'medicine' (*yi* 医 / 醫), at least in early Chinese medicine, shamans were regarded as specialists for medical questions and demons were seen as responsible for causing illnesses. Michel Strickman (2002) differentiates between "Buddhist demons" imported from India and indigenous "Daoistic demons", which over time amalgamated and built syncretic demons so that "any attempt to winnow out indigenous elements supposedly untouched by Buddhist influence may well be futile" (Strickman 2002: 68). Demons causing danger to health and even to life could emerge as animals; for example as fox, snake, dog or tiger, but also as merely immaterial returning souls of deceased relatives (ibid. 69, 74). The text 'Introduction to Medicine' from the 16th century (*Yixue Rumen* 醫學 入門) by Li Ting (李 挺) shows an illness episode caused by a demon and describes some methods to cure the possessed:

> The symptoms resulting from attack by [...] demonic influences appear in the evening or at night when one visits the latrine, goes out into the woods, wanders through empty, cold houses, or stops in places where no man has previously trod. Suddenly, demon-like beings are seen. Their evil influences enter through the nose and the mouth, and the victim falls unexpectedly to the ground. The four extremities grow cold. Both hands tighten into fists. Clear blood flows from the nose and mouth. Consciousness fades. After a short time, any help is hopeless. [...]
> Whenever someone is expectedly unable to move, all his relatives are summoned, and they stand around the victim, beating drums and lighting fires. Or musk [...] or a similar substance is burned. [..] In certain acute cases, five *qian*[24] pulverized rhinoceros horn, and one *fen*[25] each of cinnabar and musk, both also pulverized, should be taken. (*Yixue Rumen*, cited in Unschuld 1985: 217).

Up until the last two dynasties of the Chinese empire, the *Ming* (*ming chao* 明朝; 1386-1644) and the *Qing Dynasties* (*qing chao* 清朝; 1644-1911), many treatise on demonic medicine were written (Strickman 2002: 216), which reveals that not only 'ordinary people' believed in evil forces but also medical experts accounted them as etiological relevant.

---

24 Ancient Chinese measuring unit.
25 Ancient Chinese measuring unit.

Medical Pluralism and the Contemporary Situation of Chinese Medicine in China

Chinese Medicine versus Western Medicine

For millennia, Chinese medicine was unchallenged in its role as the primary and predominant medical system in China. With the introduction of contemporary Western medicine by missionaries in the 16th and 17th century, Chinese medicine was confronted with a different medical system for the first time.[26] But it was not until the groundbreaking discoveries of the late 19th and early 20th century that propelled Western medicine to the forefront, that Chinese intellectuals accused Chinese medicine of being backward or out of date. Nevertheless, the number of purely Western medical institutions was quite insignificant at the beginning of the 20th century. Between 1886 and 1929, there were only 24 private and public Western medical schools with only 3,816 graduates; a nationwide survey in 1935 found that only 5,390 doctors trained in Western medicine were practising in China, of which 1.128 had their base of activity in Shanghai (Xu 1997: 848). However, due to these low numbers of Western practitioners Chinese intellectuals were even more spurred to abandon what they thought was pure superstition. As Crozier (1965) shows, there was a clear line between the supporters of Chinese medicine and the supporters of Western medicine right between the ruling class of Republican China. On the one hand, the leading group, the *Goumindang* Party (GMD, founded in 1912), was in favour of Chinese medicine; however, the ministries and government departments, on the other hand, tried their best to abolish it and promoted Western medicine (Croizier 1965: 862). The result was a struggle between the preservers of national essence against Western imperialism and the promoters of science and modernity instead of backwardness and superstition (ibid. 875). This struggle is indicated in the different terms for Chinese and Western medicine common at that time. Western medicine simply was referred to as that – Western medicine (*xiyi* 西医), whereas Chinese medicine, according to the political standpoint, was referred to as 'ancient medicine' (*guyi* 故医), 'outdated medicine' (*jiuyi* 旧医), 'national medi-

---

26 For the early encounter of Chinese and Western medicine I refer to Linda Barnes (2007).

cine' (*guoyi* 国医) or 'Chinese medicine' (*zhongyi* 中医) (c.f. Taylor 2004 or Scheid 2006).

But not only parts of the nationalist party were sceptical towards Chinese medicine; among the members and supporters of the Chinese Communist Party (CCP, founded in 1921), there were some eager advocates of the new, Western medicine. For example Chen Duxiu (陳獨秀 / 陈独秀), one of the leaders of the May Fourth Movement27 and founding member of the CCP, accused the native doctors of being

> ignorant of science, not only unfamiliar with human anatomy, but also unable to analyse the properties of medicine. As for bacteria and contagious disease, they have never heard of them. They can only parrot-talk about five elements (Chen Duxiu, quoted in Croizier 1965: 2).

Also one the most famous writers of the republican era and opponent of the *Guomindang* (GMD) Government, Lu Xun (鲁迅 / 鲁迅)[28], polemized Chinese medicine in his well-known short story 'The Medicine' (*Yao* 藥).[29] After the victory over the GMD and the end of the civil war in 1949 one would think that a new era of Western medicine was about to dawn. But the CCP and the new government realized that, on the one hand Western trained doctors were considered as politically more dangerous and less controllable, and on the other hand they increasingly perceived the entire adoption of Western medicine as "capitalistic, imperialistic and colonialistic" (Unschuld 1979: 127). Despite this, during the Chinese civil war, Mao Zedong sought the task of updating the old medicine (i.e. Chinese medicine) with the new medicine (i.e. Western medicine) and he cast a shadow on Chinese medicine by implicitly connecting it to backward feudalism. In a speech given in October of 1944, he said: "We must tell the masses that they should wage a struggle against their own illiteracy, superstition and

---

27 The May Fourth Movement was a political movement originating from student protests in Beijing starting at May 4th, 1919.
28 Lu Xun was medically educated as he studied Medicine at the University of Sendai (Japan).
29 Although Monschein (1989) remarks that criticising the superstition of Chinese medicine is not the only intention of the author, it is clear that the blood-soaked steamed bread which is recommended as a reliable medicine against tuberculosis is intended to cast a shadow on Chinese medical beliefs.

unhygienic habits" (Mao Zedong 1953, quoted in Taylor 2001: 345-346).[30] But he also made it clear that the Chinese people cannot rely on Western medicine alone and that the "old doctors" should be educated and remoulded for the people's sake (ibid.). This process was carried out under the political catchphrases 'newness' (*xin* 新), 'science' (*kexue* 科學) and 'unity' (*tuanjie* 團結) to satisfy the medical needs of the nation (Taylor 2001: 344, also see Unschuld 2003: 259).

The term 'Traditional Chinese Medicine' (TCM) also derived from political ideas. According to Kim Taylor it first appeared in a political context in the second half of 1955 and the first publication using this term was an article by Fu Lianzhang (傅连璋)[31] in the Chinese Medical Journal in September 1955[32], the English-language announcement of the political slogan 'Doctors of Western Medicine Study Chinese Medicine' (Taylor 2005: 84). Taylor makes clear that the term TCM is foreign-specific and coined with the intention of marketing and promoting Chinese medicine for a foreign audience (ibid. 83). During my frequent stays in China, I never witnessed the use of the term TCM in Chinese (it would be *chuantong zhongyi* 传统中医); also the research literature states that this term is totally uncommon in China (for example Scheid 2006: 60 or Taylor 2004: 102). During my fieldwork, while talking with Chinese people using their mother-tongue, they referred to the topic as 'Chinese medicine' (*zhongyi* 中医), but using English they, without exception, used the term 'Traditional Chinese Medicine'.

So without hesitation, one can say that the tradition of 'Traditional Chinese Medicine' covers not more than perhaps 60 years. I therefore employ this term only in its specific meaning and use the term 'Chinese medicine' (CM), when I am referring to medical practice in China outside the biomedical paradigm and inside the Chinese paradigm of *qi*, *yin yang* and other indigenous Chinese concepts.

Taylor's (2005: 12-13) frames the encounter of Chinese and Western medicine and the official party line in the PRC under concise political slogans which is summarily useful: from 1945 to 1950 the aim was 'The Co-operation of Chinese

---

30 For this whole topic I highly recommend the publications of Kim Taylor, especially her PhD-Thesis "Chinese Medicine in Early Communist China, 1945-63" published in 2005.
31 Fu Lianzahng (1894-1968), President of the Chinese Medical Association and Deputy Minister of Health
32 Fu Lianzhang (1955): Why our Western-trained doctors should learn Traditional Chinese Medicine. Chinese Medical Journal 73 (5), 363-367.

and Western Medicines' (*zhong xi yi hezuo*中西医合作), whereas in the 1950 both the campaign for 'The Unification of Chinese and Western Medicines' (*zhong xi yi tuanjie* 中西医团结) and the campaign 'Chinese Medicine Studies Western Medicine' (*zhongyi xuexi xiyi* 中医学习西医) started. In 1954 the inverted slogan 'Western Medicine Studies Chinese Medicine' (*xiyi xuexi zhongyi* 西医学习中医) was promoted and the main paradigm starting in 1958, which is still more or less an official position, is 'The Integration of Chinese and Western Medicine' (*zhong xi yi jiehe* 中西医结合).

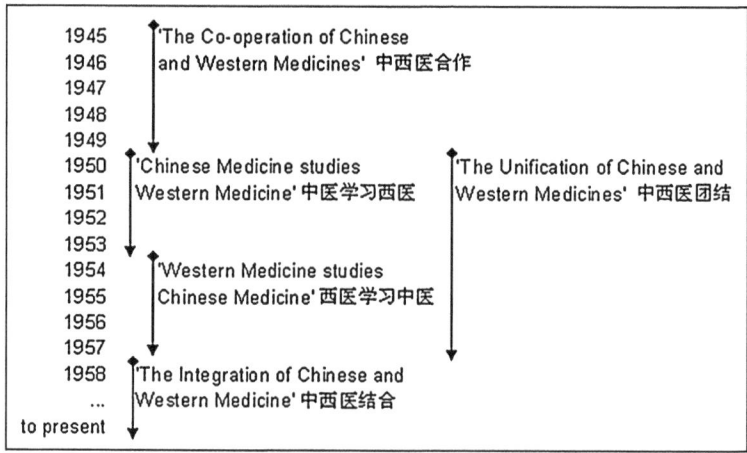

Fig. 2: Political slogans concerning the relationship between Chinese and Western medicine (c.f. Taylor 2005: 12-13).

So in a little more than ten years the notion of Chinese medicine "was moved from a marginally accepted sideline of the national health care system to an essential part of it" (Taylor 2005: 13) or, to quote Chinese politicians, from the "collected garbage of several thousand years" (Tan Zhuang, 1941) to the statement "Chinese Medicine is a great treasure house and should be dilligently explored and improved upon" (Calligraphy by Mao Zedong, 1958) (both quoted in Unschuld 1985: 251). The guideline for this transformation was a Maoist-Marxist one, with the main aim to "demonstrate national progress and raise cultural standards" (Hinrichs 1998: 293) according to the ideology of the ruling party. This inevitably led to political implications in the medical sector and imposed a political and ideological dimension on the discourse concerning Chinese medicine. Although not prohibited during the Cultural Revolution (1966-1976) and not suffering the same fate as other 'traditional' institutions which were abandoned and destroyed, the political implications of Chinese medicine caused a deep uneasiness in many people, putting it close to other 'traditional', 'superstitious' and 'feudalistic' techniques and concepts. As I will show in Chapter Seven, to this day, this has an impact on concepts and on the choosing behaviour of certain social groups.

This transformation of Chinese medicine and its firm political implications has led to a passionate discussion, especially in German scientific circles, about whether 'modern' Chinese medicine is still comparable to the pre-revolution Chinese medicine. Manfred Porkert (1973, 1976, and 1986) claimed that Chinese medicine is a coherent "system of thought" and has a tradition of some thousand years, visible in "basic standards of value" like the Five Phases or the *yin yang* dichotomy (Porkert 1976: 69-75). As Taylor (2004) shows, Porkert's sources for his idea of coherence and tradition are not classic original sources, as he claims, but are mainly derived from a text published by the Nanjing Academy of TCM in 1958; thus Porkert's study is "largely based on a 1958 text" and he is "at best under-representing and at worst mis-representing the revolutionary nature of material [he is] using" (Taylor 2004: 108).

Paul Unschuld, one of the main investigators of Chinese medicine in Germany, also disagrees with Porkert by stating that Chinese medicine has never known "one dominant school of thought" (Unschuld 1992: 54).

Volker Scheid (2002) enumerates the multiple influences on the development of Chinese medicine in the last 60 years:

> Nationalism, Maoism, valorization of science and technology, market economics, western model of rationality, the protection of the image of China as a country with profound and unbroken cultural heritage (Scheid 2002: 65).

Some of these influences, like science and technology, market economics or cultural heritage, were important to the ideas and attitudes of informants towards Chinese medicine, too. In Chapter Six, these connections will be clarified in detail.

This whole debate can be integrated in the larger ethnological discussions about "Orientalism" (Said, 1979) and the "Invention of Tradition" (Hobsbawm & Ranger 1983). At the very beginning of his influential book Orientalism, Edward Said calls the orient "almost an European invention, […] a place of romance, exotic beings, [...] and remarkable experiences" (Said 1979: 1). In this paragraph we could substitute Orient with Chinese medicine without much friction. Thomas Ots, for example, shows how Western doctors of TCM accuse their Chinese colleagues of betraying their own cultural heritage after they observed differences between classical medical texts (or at least their translations) and the clinical reality in China. Instead, these Western doctors try to conserve the "true, authentic theory of Chinese medicine" ("die wahre, authentische Theorie der Chinesischen Medizin") (Ots 1987: 185). Said describes the perceived responsibility of one 'dealing with the orient' that it is "his duty to rescue some portion of a lost, past classical Oriental grandeur in order to 'facilitate ameliorations' in the present orient" (Said 1979: 79). For Ots and for others, TCM often seems to be more an invention of the West than an collection of cultural concepts and artefact of the East. As Paul Unschuld puts it, traditional Chinese medicine "often enough, appears to mirror Western ideals of what an 'alternative' medicine should be like rather than original Chinese thought" (Unschuld 1987: 1023). In Said's terms, this truly is a "European idea of the Orient" (Said 1979: 16).33

However, as one can see in the efforts of systematize and formalize Chinese medicine and also in the invention of the term 'traditional Chinese medicine', in contrast to Said, this Chinese Orient was by no means totally powerless or dominated by the West. In the field of Chinese medicine there are many active 'Oriental' agents who actively conduct discourses concerning Chinese medicine. Already at the beginning of the encounter between Chinese and Western medicine, Chinese doctors adapted Western medical thought and techniques, such as particular surgical techniques, into Chinese medicine and thus "selectively modified their own tradition" (Andrews 1994: 159).

This modification of tradition to a certain extent complies with the conditions Eric Hobsbawm (1983) established for his idea of an "Invented Tradition". The "use of ancient material to construct invented traditions [...] for a quite

---

33   For a concise overview of the Orientalism in the work of early European China-scholars, which usually were (protestant) missionaries, see Wang 2008. Here, the author clearly outlines a "different style of Orientalism", not so much the "orient-occident dichotomy than the Christian-Heathen divide" (Wang 2008: 24). For further reference on the connection between Orientalism and Sinology see Chan 2009. I also refer to Weigelin-Schwiedrzik (2007) about the question, to which extent Asia is a European invention. Not surprisingly, the wheel spins the other way round, too, and Said has been criticized for neglecting that there is also a process of "Occidentalisation". For the Chinese case, I refer to the monography Occidentalism: Theory of counter-discourse in post Mao China (Chen 1994) and to the article Chinese History and the question of Orientalism (Dirlik 1996a).

novel purpose" and the question of "how far they [i.e. the 'inventers'] may be forced to invent new languages or devices, or extend the old symbolic vocabulary beyond its established limits" (Hobsbawm 1983: 6-7) goes together with the considerations of the people in charge of modernizing Chinese medicine and thereby 'creating' TCM according to the official party line. By keeping old concepts like *qi* and *yin yang*, combining them with socialist ideological concepts like dialectics and manifesting them in institutions in the shape of socialist work-units (*danwei* 单位) (c.f. Hsu 1999: 8), TCM clearly adheres to Hobsbawm's conditions of 'invented tradition'.[34]

The Contemporary Situation of Chinese Medicine

For Scheid, the contemporary Chinese medicine is by no means a totality, because "the visible pluralities of Chinese medicine [...] are not reducible to a singular cultural logic or process of cultural production" (Scheid 2002: 13). He describes the non-ideological habit of doctors of Chinese medicine in switching between the demarcation-lines of Chinese and Western medicine (ibid. 158), a case also witnessed throughout this research. Chinese doctors make use of examination methods, therapies or drugs derived from Western medicine and have no problems synchronizing them with Chinese medical thought.35

In contemporary China, at least in the big cities, there are a variety of different medical offerings to choose from; due to the opening policy, growing of markets and the processes of globalization and internationalization, a marketplace for medicines has emerged in the last decade which is still growing and diversifying. Of course the choice is limited to the economic condition. But with market reforms, the old health care system was condemned to a slow extinction. Up until the early 1980s, the population was covered by one of several types of insurance schemes: the 'Government Insurance Scheme' for employees of the state-run enterprises; the 'Labour Insurance Scheme' for the urban population; and the 'Cooperative Medical Scheme' for the rural population (Ramesh & Wu

---

34 For a closer look on invented tradition and Chinese medicine I particularly refer to Martha Hanson 1997, 1998.
35 An interesting and early example of this plurality is cited by Bridie Andrews (1994: 153), where she reports about an article written in a Chinese journal in 1909 dealing with the diagnosis and treatment of 'malaria'. The article's author, a Chinese physician called Lin Xiangeng (林先耕), mixed without hesitation Chinese concepts like qi with western concepts like nerves.

2009: 2257; also see Ho 1995: 1065). This system broke down in the 1990s. The state-owned enterprises as well as the collective farms were dismantled and with these institutions, the medical care they provided faded away, too. Additionally, the financial situation of the public health care sector grew more and more difficult (Ramesh & Wu 2009: 2257). Many reforms to privatize and decentralize the health care institutions were carried out and although the government drastically reduced financial support for the health care system, it still controls prices on common drugs in order to avoid dramatic price increases (Xu & Yang 2009: 134). Nevertheless, almost 50% of the Chinese health expenditures in 2006 were out of pocket payments, whereas 18% were government health expenditures and 32% social health expenditures (Xu et al. 2011: 205). Currently, there are three major insurance schemes in China: firstly the 'New Cooperative Medical Scheme', a voluntary scheme which is intended to cover the rural population; secondly, the 'Basic Medical Insurance Scheme' which is mandatory for urban employees and retirees; and finally, the 'Urban Resident Scheme' which is a voluntary scheme for children, students and urban residents without income (ibid. 205).

Western medicine plays a dominant role in the Chinese heath system. In 2003, a survey discovered that more than 50% of the doctors in Chinese health clinics practised Western medicine, more than 32% practised both Western and Chinese medicine while less than 18% practised Chinese medicine alone (Xu & Yang 2009: 135).[36] The numbers of health professionals practising Chinese medicine has been on the decline in the last few years, from approximately 350.000 doctors in 1997 to approximately 250.000 in 2006 (ibid. 205). But one has to take into account that there are different levels of institutionalization of Chinese medicine and that there exists "Chinese medicine beyond the institution" (Farquhar 1994a: 19).

---

36 Interestingly this correlates with very similar answering patterns I discuss in chapter 6. Looking at the choosing behaviour of urban residents, there, too, was a domination of Western medical institutions, followed by the institutions providing combined medicine, while pure Chinese medical institutions only ended third.

Excursion: Ethnology and Emotions

Although the emotions as perceived in Chinese society and their perception as relevant in medical terms, especially as potential pathogenic, are an important part of my work, I neither looked for the "discovery of the culture-specific distinctiveness of emotional behaviour", nor tried to reveal "how emotions are shaped by cultural factors", which Röttger-Rössler (2002: 147) defines as the main assignment of ethnology in the investigation of emotions. Nevertheless, I try to outline a short overview of the emotions as investigated by ethnology, because there are some connections to my research.

Since the European ancient times, human emotions have been on the agenda of the Western philosophic and scientific community. The ancient Greek philosophers spent a good amount of time thinking about human emotions and created very persistent ideas and models. For example, Plato (428/427 B.C. – 348/347 B.C.) identified the trio Reason, Passion and Desire as a suitable description of the human mind, a classification which is still prevailing in modern Philosophy and Psychology, albeit the terminology has changed to Cognition, Emotion and Motivation. Besides this trio, the dualistic view of Rene Descartes (1596-1650) was and still is efficacious. He imagined human as a combination of a body, which is machine-like and functions for the, in his view, more important mind. This mind is what distinguishes human from animal as well as gives the option of rational thinking and free will thus connecting the human being to God. For Descartes, it is obvious that the mind is the part that makes human beings distinctively human as the body is nothing without the mind.[37] For example if humans perceive a dry throat, it is the mind that tells the human being that he or she is thirsty and should drink water. The purely mechanical action of the body is complemented by the mind's idea about the human need to drink (Descartes, cited in Burkitt 1999: 7-11).

---

37 Neuroscientist's extensive critique on Descartes' dualistic view can only be referred to very briefly: Antonio Damasio describes this dualistic perception and its modern reshaping –the mind being the software running in a piece of hardware called brain (248) – as "Descartes' Error" (1994) and claims that feelings "depend on a dedicated multi-component system that is indissociable from biological regulation" and postulates a "connecting trail [...] from reason to feelings to body" (245). LeDoux argues in favour of the "neural basis of emotions" (1995: 208) and ultimately identifies the "Emotional Brain" (1996). All these critics have in common that they emphasize the biological functioning of the brain in dealing with emotional arousal.

This paradigm, rising from a Christian, central-European school of thought, had far reaching impacts for different parts of sciences and humanities as well as ethnological research. In early years of ethnology, it was used as a distinction tool for non-European societies to differentiate between the 'cultivated, rational and civilized Europeans' and the 'wild, irrational and uncivilized savage' in order to determine the demeanour of people at the outmost border of humankind or even beyond. As ethnology of the 19th and 20th century went hand in hand with nationalism and colonialism and furthermore claimed to be based on empirical verifiable facts whereas emotions where defined as 'wild' and 'irrational', the ethnologists of that time mostly avoided investigating the emotions (Svasek 2005: 2-3).

In 1935, Marcel Mauss wrote his book *La Techniques du Corps* and manifested the perception of the body being a tool that can be utilized in different, culturally determined ways. The 'culture and personality' school of theory of the 1930s and 40s, founded by Franz Boas' disciples Margaret Mead and Ruth Benedict, focused en passant on emotions. Benedict's *Patterns of Culture* (1934) postulates a connection between the personality of the individual and a specific cultural pattern of the whole group. Margaret Mead (1928, 1930, and 1935) tried to demonstrate how personalities of grown ups are formed during culturally specific forms of socialisation. The "emotional turn" (Röttger-Rössler 2004: 2) in the 1970s and 1980s has led to increasing interest in emotions in relation to culture. The body was no longer only perceived as a tool; multiple 'body concepts' were developed in which different levels of social and societal interaction completed the picture of human beings as consisting of bodies and emotions. The idea of "Two Bodies": the "physical body" and a "social body", was groundbreaking for Mary Douglas (1970). Several years later, Nancy Scheper-Hughes and Margaret Lock (1987) identified "Three Bodies": the "individual body", the "social body" and the "body politic". Barely a decade ago, Elisabeth Hsu (2003) postulated as to whether or not there are really three bodies, or perhaps even four (*"Die drei Körper – oder sind es vier?"*).

In the last decades, ethnological research involving human emotions, the management of emotions and the connection to other parts of culture has increasingly become popular. Despite the infancy of the concepts of emotion and culture connections having passed, current discourse in ethnological research concerning the subject is still influenced by the ideas of Descartes. One can divide the ethnologists working on this subject into the two categories which Descartes imagined 350 years ago: one group mainly focuses on the body and the biology, whereas the other group mainly focuses on the mind and the culture. On the one hand, there is a biological-universalistic approach which defines emotions as a primarily biological entity. This approach concedes that culture is important in the way that it influences emotions and inducts variety, but it identifies a set of emotions which is some kind of 'biological raw material' and therefore not culture-specific. Culture's part is to carve this 'raw material' into specific end products. On the other hand, adherents to the so-called constructivist approach emphasize the idea of emotions as primarily culture-based. Culture-specific appraisals and evaluations of situations are the starting point of emotional activity and the physiological arousal is only a reaction and therefore secondary (Röttger-Rössler 2002: 147-148).

Emotions as "Complex Reactions in the Struggle of Survival" (Plutchick 1982: 551)

Taking a closer look at the first mentioned approach, the biological-universalistic entails that the researcher's main interest is on looking for a set of basic emotions which are common for all human beings. Different works, especially by Paul Ekman (for example 1972, 1981, and 1984), partly in cooperation with Wallace Friesen (for example 1969 and 1975) as well as works by Caroll Izard (1971 and 1977) and other researchers showed that different people, no matter what cultural background they had, could identify some certain facial expressions and connect them to emotions. Ekman and Friesen condensed these results in a set of six basic emotions: happiness, surprise, fear, anger, disgust, and sadness (Ekman, Friesen & Sorenson 1969, Ekman & Friesen 1975).[38] As there can be no doubt concerning the culturally specific characteristics of emotional expressions, they developed the concept of "display rules", a culturally imparted knowledge which allows the individual to behave and express emotions in a culturally adequate manner (see Röttger-Rössler 2004: 12-18).

This "traditional theory of the emotions" (Bedford 1986: 15) anchors the origin of emotions in phylogenesis. Rooted deep down in the genetic code, some reactions to certain stimuli like threat help in the evolutionary struggle of survival.

---

38 For a broader overview of the concept of 'Basic Emotions', I refer to volume with the same name edited by Stein & Oatley (1992).

This leads to impulsive actions like the fight or flight instinct. The emotional experience is inseparably connected to bodily sensations; for example to an increased heart beat rate, to the blushing of the face, to the rising of the neck hair, among others. These bodily sensations are a preparation for the anticipated scenario which follows the threat, either fight or flight. Neurophysiology has contributed to this by showing that during some emotional experiences, the limbic system of the human brain is active, whereas during other emotional sensations, the frontal lobe is involved. The limbic system mainly is involved in emotions which are labelled as 'instinctive' and 'basic' such as fear (Casimir 2009a: 70), while the frontal lobe is active during emotional episodes which are seen as culturally influenced and shaped, like shame or envy (Lupton 1998: 12). Evolutionary psychology therefore assesses emotion as an advantage in evolution, not only for the single individual (fugue or the preparation to fight as a reaction to fear or threat etc.), but also as an advantage for a whole group or even society (compassion in a state of emergency, mutual confidence, etc.). Plutchik (1982: 550) writes:

> When a survival-related emergency situation arises, emotions act try to re-establish the conditions that existed before the situation arose. For example, if a threat occurs, the individual's fear directs him to carry out actions that will eliminate the threat and reduce the fear.

Ulich (1992: 36) summarizes the positions of the biological approach:

> Während einerseits phylogenetisch entstandene, genetisch festgelegte und überlebensdienliche Grundemotionen allen Menschen gemeinsam sind, so müssen andererseits für deren Auslöser und Kontrolle im Laufe der individuellen Entwicklung in einer bestimmten Kultur doch auch bestimmte Lernprozesse stattfinden.[39]

Just like Ulich, other social scientists see the importance of culture as a factor in emotional reaction. For Appadurai (1990: 93) "emotions are discursive publics forms" as well as "universal biological substrate", and Casimir (2009b: 288) reminds us to "distinguish between the basic biological 'innate' part and the learned culture- or group-specifically coded behavioural component(s)". But

---

39 "While on the one hand, phylogenetically originated, genetically determined basic emotions are common to all people, on the other hand, for triggering and control, there must be learning process in individual evolution in one's culture" (my translation).

whereas the advocates of the biological approach concede culture to diversify emotions on the grounds of biologically rooted basic emotions, other approaches emphasise the role of culture as foundation and constitution of emotions.

Emotions as "Embodied Thought" (Rosaldo 1984: 143)

The differentiation in the two layers; biological founded basic emotions and culturally grounded variation in displaying emotions, elicited some objections. Robert Solomon, for example, speaks of "hopeless simplification" (Solomon 1981: 250) and insists that emotions neither can be separated from culture-specific interpretative system nor from their biological roots. They are part of both worlds. Catherine Lutz criticises the categories which where build to classify emotions as merely unreflecting ethno-centric concepts which cannot be used in the analysis of non-Western societies (Lutz 1988: 42).

As an alternative to avoid the model of the two layers as well as the suspected ethno-centric bias, some researchers promote a constructivist approach to "separate emotions from their physiological determination" and to "locate them in the cognitive dimension" (Röttger-Rössler 2004: 46). Exemplarily, Catherine Lutz is to be named as a representative of this approach due to her far-reaching work and publications (for example 1986, 1988, 1996; with White 1986; with Abu-Lughod 1990). She criticises that from a Western perspective, emotions are frequently seen as natural in contradiction to cultural, as irrational in contradiction to rational, as chaotic in contradiction to organised and as physical in contradiction to intellectual; emotions became a "disadvantaged contrast to more valued personal processes, particularly to cognition or rational thought" (Lutz 1996: 151). Instead she demands that "cultural formulations of emotions" are to be studied in their genuine social context which would make a much better contribution to the research on the public, social and cognitive dimensions of emotional experience (Lutz & White 1986: 429).

For the constructivist approach, Röttger-Rössler (2004: 45) summarises five important assumptions:

1. Emotions are situational appraisals on the foundation of culture-specific moral concepts and beliefs; therefore they are subject to cognitive processes.
2. The experience of emotions is based on learned norms, values and aims, which work as a pattern for interpretation. Emotions determine and define

experience. At the same time, emotions reduce complexity as they allow connecting different situations to same emotional appraisal.
3. Emotions are socially compulsory reactions. An individual has to show emotions in certain contexts to establish contact to the cultural nexus of the group.
4. In opposition to the assumption of uncommitted passions, constructivist approaches assume emotions to be purposeful and targeted. They are always related to events, people or things and are not irrational phenomena.
5. Due to the close connection to the value system, emotions contain important social functions. Group members are motivated to behave according to values and norms of the group, which leads to a "positive" emotional feedback.

Of course the constructivist approach elicited critique as well. Especially criticised was the high level of construction and therefore a principal impossibility to compare emotional utterances. Lyon (1998: 43) writes:

> While accepting that the cultural dimensions of emotions are an important subject of inquiry, wholly constructionist approaches can obscure our view of the phenomenon of emotion in the larger sense, that is, the understanding of the importance of emotion not only in culturally produced and mediated experience, but in social and bodily agency as conceived in terms of its foundation in social structure.

Bridging the gap between the biological-universalistic and the cultural-constructivist approaches is the aim of the "social cognitive neuroscience" (Ochser & Lieberman 2001: 719) respectively of the "cultural neuroscience" (Seligman & Brown 2010: 130). They emphasize the influence of social or cultural impact not only to the evaluation of processes or to the execution of culture-specific display rules, but also directly to the operation processes of the brain. Consequently, emotions are not only automatic responses to certain stimuli but are subject to controlling attention and cognitively changing of meanings (Ochser & Gross 2005: 242).

For Rainer Schützeichel (2006), social science developed two additional approaches to this field. First, phenomenological theories place special emphasis on the bodily experience of emotions; not the "objectified", scientifically analysed and verifiable dimension, but the emotional experience is the important reference. In ethnology, this approach is deeply shaped by studies following the "embodiment theory" (Csordas 1990). The "lived body" (Nettleton & Watson

1998: 9) shows the inescapability "of being human as being a body" (Csordas 1994: 3) and does not allow for the separation of the physical and the mental reactions to emotional appraisals.[40]

Secondly, in an attempt for synthesis, Schützeichel introduces a multi-component theory which incorporates physical and cognitive processes as well as subjective experience. Mees (2006: 107) states more precisely that this approach encompasses cognitive, motivational, expressive, and psycho-physiological dimension of emotions without neglecting subjective emotional experience. Although all-encompassing, this approach seems to be quite ineffective due to its inherent broadness.

---

40 See also the work of Feldman (1991) investigating the "Narrative of the Body and Political Terror in Northern Ireland", of Scheper-Hughes (1992) about "The Violence of Everyday Life in Brazil" and of Winkler (1994) analysing "Rape Trauma".

2. Research Questions and Methodology

As already pointed out in the introduction, I detect a gap in the present scientific literature on Chinese medicine in mainland China. In the existing ethnographies, it has been clearly ascertained that there are different medical systems in China. Aside from Western-style biomedicine, there is an institutionalised Chinese medicine which refers to a certain continuity of indigenous concepts which is also open for innovations. Outside of institutions and much more informal but nonetheless accepted and practiced, there is another sector of indigenous health care (see Farquhar 1994a and Hsu 1999). However, these studies, indispensable as they are, in the majority of cases do not focus on lay people and their attitudes towards Chinese medicine, Western medicine, or other medical systems. At present, no detailed study has been conducted to analyse whether there is a comparable division on the potential patient's side, whether Western biomedicine has become a formative medical worldview, whether indigenous concepts still prevail, whether there is a third direction or whether there is a mixture of different concepts. It can be expected that different social agents have certain attitudes towards different medical systems or treatments; we do not know whether older urban residents are more or less open to Chinese medicine than younger people or what young white-collar workers think of acupuncture and herbal drugs, about Western psychotherapy or other biomedical treatments. Furthermore, we can not see if women and men are using Chinese or Western medicine in different, gender-related ways. Consequently, I ask questions about the concepts of illness and health in urban China and investigate the ways in which Beijing inhabitants utilize these concepts

Basically I am seeking to answer the question of whether indigenous ideas are still prevailing in Chinese urban society, if they are removed by Western dominated ideas of the biomedical system or if there originated a mixture of ideas out of different medical systems. Going more into detail, the 'Seven Emotions'[41] should be focused on. Do these 'Seven Emotions' play an important role concerning health and illness in everyday life? Is there measurable knowledge concerning the interaction between emotions and health? Does this knowledge coincide with theories written in the classics, in modern textbooks or other written sources? Why are certain concepts concerning the interface of emotion and health more popular than others? Do people see the influence of emotions on health and illness? How do certain urban agents make use of Chinese or Western

---

41   See chapter 1.

medicine? Are there different attitudes and choices related to gender, age, education or economical situation?

Methods

The research is divided into two main sections. The first part is a quintessential analysis of the relationship between emotions and health in different texts related to Chinese Medicine. I analyse some chosen passages of ancient, classicphilosophical texts as well as medical classics, but also give an introduction to recent medical textbooks and outline their assertions regarding these questions. Furthermore, I discuss as a sideline the research literature on Chinese emotionality, emphasizing psychological literature, for example by Kleinman & Lin (1980) or Bond (1987, 1993).

The second section will consist of data collected during the fieldwork in Beijing and its analysis. This fieldwork was separated into three periods totalling eight months. In March and April of 2008 I was in Beijing for two months to establish first contacts and to explore whether the research concept was practical; a small pre-test of a preliminary questionnaire was conducted to estimate the willingness of potential interviewees to talk about this topic. The main fieldwork was done in Summer of 2010, when I returned to Beijing for four months to conduct the survey. In March and April of 2011, I finalized my data gathering by conducting interviews, both informal with survey participants and formal with medical experts.

Consequently, my data consists of both quantitative and qualitative components. For the quantitative data, I created a questionnaire survey comprising 47 questions (see appendix 1); the variables consist of dichotomic variables like 'yes-or-no' questions and of polytomic variables, where the informants could choose between different possible answers. Furthermore, I used an item-battery, where the informants would respond whether they agree with or reject certain statements concerning Chinese medicine. Additionally, there are some questions with open answers. For statistics, I collected data on gender, age, occupation, income, education and ethnicity. After a small-scale pre-test at the very beginning of my fieldwork period, which revealed some minor weaknesses and led to a revision of the questionnaire, the survey was carried out in residential neighbourhoods in the city centre of Beijing, in so called 'small neighbourhoods' or *xiaoqu* (小区), where I asked people living in this area if they were willing to participate in my questionnaire. These neighbourhoods were all located inside the 4th ring road (see Fig. 4).[42]

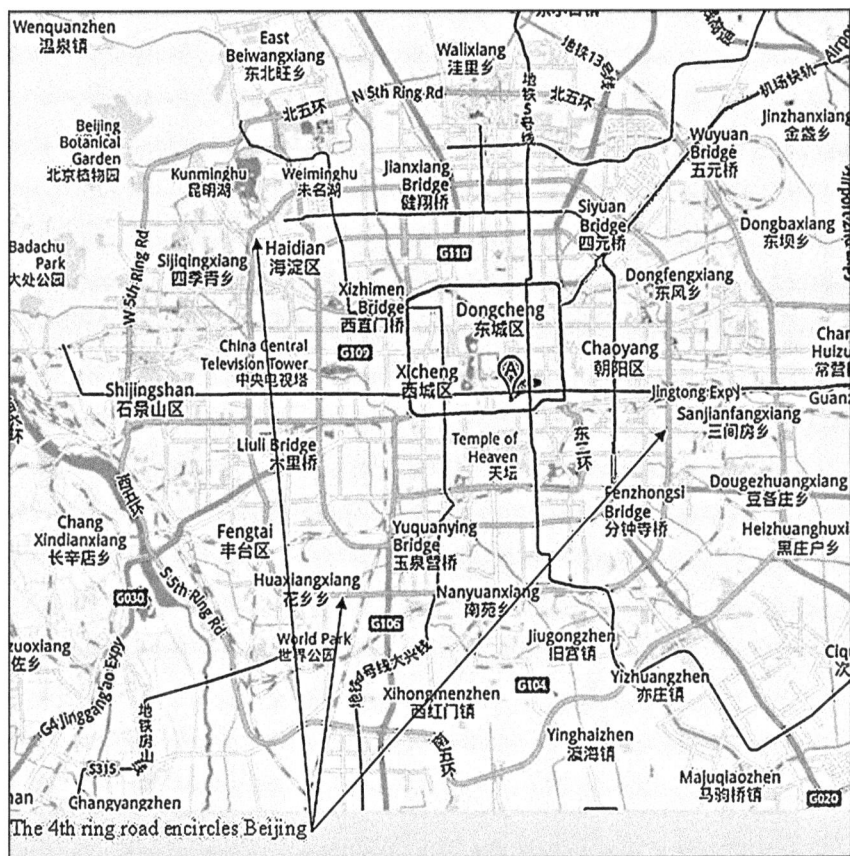

Fig. 3: Map of the city centre of Beijing with the 4th ring road (Google maps, own modifications).

---

42 The vast territory of Beijing is commonly divided into circles according to ring roads. The 1st ring road encircles the Forbidden City, the 2nd ring road follows the course of the ancient city walls and its route is the same as the subway line 2. Between the 3rd and the 4th ring road there is among other sites the main site of the Olympic Games 2008 and the campuses of the big universities like Beijing University (Beijing Daxue 北京大学) or Qinghua University (Qinghua Daxue 清华大学).

Together, with my colleagues from the Institute for Ethnology of the Central University for Nationalities, and in agreement with local contacts, I chose five different sites in which to conduct the survey; these sites were chosen because they represent different social groups. In the north-western part, one site was in the *Haidian* District (海淀区), in an area where modern high-rise buildings were very common as well as older compounds of five to six storey buildings. This is an area where one could expect a mixed group of residents ranging from the upper-middle class living in the modern highrises to the lower-middle class and slightly poorer residents living in the older and more rundown quarters. A second site was located in the *Fengtai* District (丰台区) in the south-west of the city, representing the residents of living quarters in close proximity to the subway station *Liujiayo* (刘家窑站), which some of the informants named as the label of this neighbourhood. Modern highrises were almost totally absent in this area whereas older six storey brick buildings or older multi-storey buildings dominate the area. Here one can expect lower-middle class inhabitants.[43] As a third site, I choose the area around the bell tower (*zhonglou* 钟楼) and the drum tower (*gulou* 鼓楼) in the *Dongcheng* District (东城区), identifiable through the street *Gulou dajie* (鼓楼大街), in the very centre of the city, a quarter which was even central in the ancient Imperial City. This is one of the last quarters which is characterized by the classic Beijing courtyard house. These areas are commonly referred to as *Hutong* (胡同) and labelled 'traditional', even if this particular neighbourhood is not far away from the prominent and booming quarter around the 'Rearward Lake' (*Houhai* 后海), an area which teems with bars and restaurants and a famous entertainment district in Beijing. Fourthly, to represent a wealthier, middle-aged upper class in my study, I choose the *Chaoyang* District (朝阳区), especially the area close to the *Guomao* Bridge (国贸桥) in the east of the city. This area is Beijing's central business district and one of the most expensive places in the city centre, almost completely covered by modern multi-storey business and apartment buildings. The fifth site contradicted the principles of choosing pure residential sites, because the *Zhongguancun* (中关村) shopping mall in the northern part of Beijing, located in the *Haidian* District (海淀区) is a huge shopping complex. It is very popular with younger people and attracts foot traffic from other parts of the city; customers come here either to shop or just to walk around and admire the range of items as well as take part

---

43 But one has to keep in mind that even this more ordinary neighbourhood without modern apartment towers is still a privileged living quarter in Beijing because it is close to the city centre and is well connected to infrastructure like main streets and public transport; therefore, poor residents and low class inhabitants are unlikely to be found in these central urban quarters.

in the busy and *'renao'* 热闹 (lit. 'hot and boisterous') atmosphere. Therefore, this site was chosen especially with regard to younger, 'modern' and 'urbanized' people.

Initially I planned to ask the informants to take the questionnaire and a ballpoint pen and fill them out by themselves. But right from the beginning of my research, I realized that this method was not feasible. Informants did not want to fill out the questions on their own; rather, they wanted me to read out the questions and then write down the answers myself. Therefore, I changed my method slightly and used the questionnaire as a foundation and structure for guided interviews, applying some "soft interview techniques" (Diekmann 2009: 440) like explaining a question or nodding in order to encourage the informants to answer. This proved advantageous because not only did I receive answers to my questions which I directly noted in the blank gaps of the questionnaire, but animated conversations arose, which encouraged other people around to take part in the conversation or to agree to also doing a questionnaire interview. Because many of my informants took their time and due to the conversations between the informants and me and among themselves, the whole procedure of completing one questionnaire took significantly more time than planned. However, by engaging in these extended conversations, they provided me with extra data which I collected by writing memory minutes. So not only did I collect a good number of verbal statements which help me to clarify some otherwise very vague positions, this quantitative questioning supplied me with a set of data which is comparable due to the structure of the questionnaire and which builds the foundation of the analysis in chapter 7.

The target group (*Grundgesamtheit*) for my survey sample was the population of Beijing[44]; I took my sample according to birth cohort and gender so that every generation as well as genders are represented in the sample. While in the younger age groups and among the oldest participants women are slightly overrepresented in the sample, men are slightly overrepresented in the middle age groups. In total, this survey had a negligibly higher number of women who took part in the survey, from 253 participants, 134 were female and 119 were male (Fig. 4).

---

44 However, no individual younger than 20 years is in my sample.

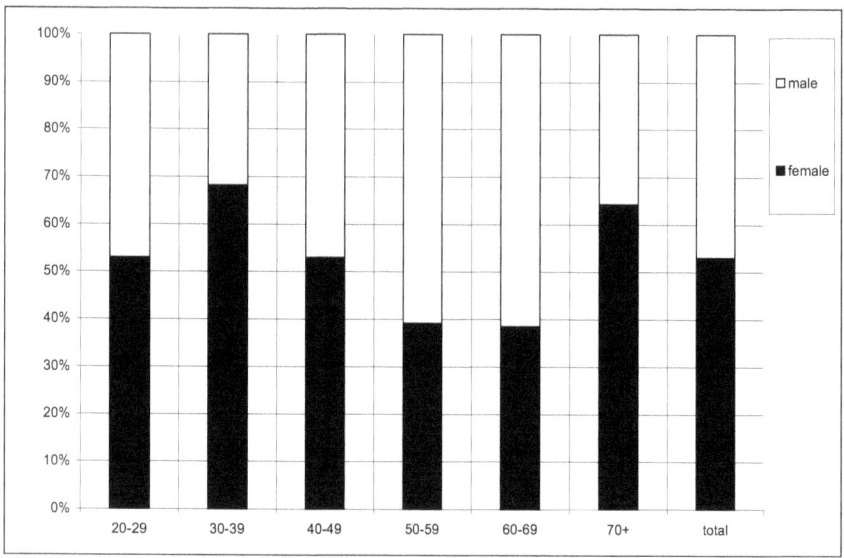

Fig. 4: Distribution of gender in age groups among survey participants (Böke: Fieldwork 20102011).

Already during the first evaluation of the survey material, I realized that there are certain specific differences in the answers of different social groups. I identified these differences on three dimensions including age, gender and educational background. This influenced my plans concerning the interviews with practitioners of Chinese medicine. Additionally, I conducted several semi-structured interviews with different experts in Chinese medicine to obtain qualitative material. However, I not only asked for the professional view on the connection between emotions and health, but also questioned the medical experts in order to find out whether their estimations would support my findings in the survey: that there can be detected a specific answering behaviour of certain social groups, and what explanations they have for this observation.[45] These queries led to an extension of my interview roadmap, shifting the impact away from the professional explanation of emotions as agents giving rise to illnesses to the question of why certain social groups use medical concepts or treatments according to Chinese medicine in specific way in which other groups do not.

---

45 According to Flick (2010), this collecting of "context information" is one of the main functions of expert interviews and allows the triangulation of different perspectives on the same topic (Flick 2010: 214-218).

Fortunately, several doctors and other clinic staff were very helpful and agreed to be interviewed; exactly 20 comprehensive interviews were collected, 12 with doctors of Chinese medicine aged between 24 and 51 years, four with students of Chinese medicine at the Beijing University of Chinese medicine (*Beijing Zhongyiyao Daxue* 北京中医药大学), three with seasoned hospital staff working in this position, and one interview with a manager of a mid-size clinic. I visited three clinics in the city centre respectively in the near suburbs of Beijing, ranging from a small size clinic to a large and famous hospital. The first, small clinic mainly treats disorders which would be biomedically denoted as stress-related or psychosomatic by using solely acupuncture and moxibustion and focusing on a middle class clientele. The second clinic is a mid-size clinic which is open to a broader public and where different "well known doctors"[46] had their weekly consultation hours. It was supplied with a pharmacy selling Chinese medicines. The well-known larger hospital is one of the main treatment and research institutions of Chinese medicine in whole China. Furthermore, I took part in a lay-person's class on illness prevention. All these participant observations, the interviews and the visits enable me not only to embellish my data with pertinent citations, which is an often expressed accusation of empirical qualitative data (Flick 2010: 488), but by slightly shifting the direction of the questions, these observations and interviews substantially support my findings and corroborate my conclusions.

Although one may read about the restrictions of doing ethnological fieldwork in China, being under suspicion or control by governing authorities or facing other difficulties due to the political system currently in power in China (for example see Hansen 2008, Thøgersen 2008), I encountered no problems conducting my fieldwork the way I wanted and planned; I always felt welcome and supported. My interviewees were very open and had no problem in addressing 'critical' points. However, due to the fact that my research topic was not politically or socially controversial, really precarious affairs were not part of the conversations. Hence, with the exception of one medical student, everyone allowed me to record their interviews.

The same is true for the participants of the survey. Of course not everyone approached on the street participated, but I estimate that approximately every fifth or sixth person asked to do the questionnaire helped me and answered my questions openly. This is an astonishingly high number and I am keen that this is

---

46 As the manager of the clinic proudly told me (Interview with the manager of Clinic B; Böke: Fieldwork 2010/2011).

due to my appearance, a europeen, blond guy walking around in solely residential areas where normally no tourist or business trip traveller will walk. Although this might have seemed quite odd for some of the residents, I never felt any distrust or rejection; instead many people reacted with curiosity.

The interaction with other ethnologists, mainly based at the 'Institute of Ethnology' of the Central University for Nationalities' (*Zhongyang Minzu Daxue*中央民族大学), was also without any restrictions or bureaucratic obstacles and they supported me and my project as far as they could.

Accordingly I have the best reason to believe that my data is trustworthy and not influenced by any political views or ideologies others than the ones wittingly or unwittingly expressed by my informants.

3. Emotions and Health in Classical Chinese Texts

The Han-Dynasty philosopher and poet Yang Xiong (扬雄, 53 BC – 18 AD) remarked that "one's writing is the picture of one's heart" (*shu xin hua ye* 书心花也), which means that one can "derive information from old documents" regarding emotions as lived experiences, reactions, and expressions (Santangelo 2003:51-52). Fortunately there is a vast amount of philosophical as well as medical literature descended from ancient times in China. One groundbreaking event in this context was the excavation of the Mawangdui (馬王堆 / 马王堆) tomb. This archaeological site, located in the city of Changsha in Hunan Province, consists of three tombs dated to the time of the Western Han-Dynasty (206 BC – 9 AD) and was excavated between 1972 and 1974. The archaeologists discovered silk fabrics covered with different texts, so far unknown or lost philosophical treatise as well as several silk bundles with medical texts; all of which date to the second century BC or older.[47] Unschuld and Ma estimate that since these times up until the dismissal of the emperor in 1911, more than 3.000 medical texts remained accessible, which covers a broad spectrum of medical knowledge (Unschuld & Ma 1984: 7).[48]

In the following chapter, I will analyse a few of these texts, both philosophical and medical, although I am well aware of certain limitations. First, there is the limitation of space and scope in the frame of an ethnological inquiry which is mainly based on empirical data. The analysis of these texts is intended, on the one hand, to serve as a possibility for comparison with my recent empirical findings and, on the other hand, it should clarify the connections between emotions and illness in the philosophical and medical history of Chinese thought which until today, as I like to show, is still formative for many parts of Chinese society. Second, although I am able to deal with texts written in classical Chinese, it may well be that I infringe certain fundamentals of sinological text analysis. For example, I can only briefly investigate terms and texts diachronic, most of my view on these classical texts is synchronic, which obviously ignores the history

---

47   For a translation and commentary of the excavated documents see Harper 1998.
48   In 1995, Unschuld speaks of 13.000 medical texts preserved until 1912 and many more lost texts (Unschuld 1995: 21). However, it is undoubted that China is equipped with a long history and an extensive corpus of medical literature.

of certain concepts[49]. But I think, for the scope of this dissertation, it is acceptable and furthermore I witnessed that my Chinese informants used the same synchronic view when they referred to, for example, the HDNJ. As my study is based on recent evaluations and findings of certain Chinese medical concepts collected among the Chinese urban population, I think it is justifiable to approach the classical texts, although I only cursory consider editorial work or change in notions on some specific terms.

Classical Philosophical Texts

The knowledge of philosophical treatises was a requirement for an upward mobility in pre-modern China and examinations for entering higher positions (*keju* 科举) in administration mainly consisted of the recitation and discussion of passages from the classic canon of Chinese philosophy.[50]

I divided this subchapter according to the two main philosophical schools, Confucianism and Daoism. Of course there are more schools of thought in Chinese history, such as Legalism or Mohism. However, Confucianism and Daoism are the most influential philosophies and are still important in modern urban China. Political and socital agents claim the importance of these schools and emphasize the tradition of these Chinese philosophies. Consequently, I can make my point by concentrating only on Confucianism and Daoism.

All these philosophical schools emerged from the politically unstable but nevertheless formative eras of Chinese philosophy termed the 'Spring and Autumn Period' (*Chunqiu shidai* 春秋时代, 722-482 BC) and the 'Warring States Period' (*Zhanguo shidai* 战国时代, 481-221 BC), sometimes summarized under the name "Hundred Schools of Thought" (*Zhuzi Baijia* 諸子百家).

---

49 For instance I refer to the discussion (Santangelo 1999, Graham 1990) about the term qing 情 and whether it can be translated as 'emotion' in texts earlier than the Han-Dynasty (i.e. before 206 BC).

50 The classical canon of Chinese philosophy comprised the 'Five Classics', i.e. Book of Change (Yijing 易經), Book of Poetry (Shijing 詩經), Classic of Documents (Shujing 書經), Book of Rites (Liji 禮記) and the Spring and Autumn Annals (Chunqiu 春秋), and the 'Four Books', i.e. The Great Learning (Da Xue 大學), The Analects of Confucius (Lunyu 論語), the Doctrine of the Mean (Zhongyong 中庸) and Mencius (Mengzi 孟子). They were chosen and compiled by the Neo-Confucian scholar Zhu Xi (1130-1200) during the Song-Dynasty.

Evidently, these philosophical schools are not monolithic blocks. Ever since their foundation[51], commentaries and modification were implemented and the thoughts of certain schools were promoted to be state doctrine, and thus faced new challenges. The Qin-Dynasty (Q*in chao* 秦朝 ; 221 BC – 207 BC) chose Legalism, whereas the succeeding Han-Dynasty (*Han chao*漢朝 / 汉朝 ; 202 BC – 220 AD) chose Confucianism. The latter became the main philosophical school in ancient China on a political and social level and was noticeably renewed and extended as Neo-Confucianism during the Song-Dynasty (*Song chao*宋朝 ; 960-1279); it has since enjoyed a revival in modern China during the last decade as Confucianism was banned during the Cultural Revolution. All of these schools also had to deal with Buddhism[52], but especially Daoism was demonstrably influenced by this new worldview, giving way for the implementation of Buddhist ideas creating a syncretic Daoism. The involvement of these two worldviews included controversy and opposition as well as syncretism (c.f. Zürcher 2007: 288-331).

All of these Chinese philosophical schools, clearly due to the experience of centuries of war and chaos, have in common that they want to achieve harmony and equilibrium as an ultimate goal. Furthermore, they fear excess in general and emotional excess in particular, as it is conceived to be dangerous and threatening to the aim of establishing harmony (Santangelo 2005: 406).

However, the two schools of Confucianism and Daoism use completely divergent approaches to achieve harmony and avoid emotional excess. Whereas Confucianism claims that emotionality is only acceptable in the framework of strict moral norms or ritual instructions in order to avoid chaos, Daoism designates this normative foundation of emotionality as hollow and aspires to "return to the original and to recover the nature", meaning to reject the "things which came into being […] but to change direction and return to its root in tranquillity and emptiness" (Xiang 2008: 503). I demonstrate these divergent paths in the following paragraphs, starting with an outline of Confucian text dealing with emotionality, followed by an analysis of analogous Daoist texts.

---

51 As Smith (2003) outlines, these different philosophical schools did not recognize themselves as schools or any form of institution in the first place. He holds that the first classification of distinct philosophical schools can be identified in the work of Han-Dynasty astrologer Sima Tan (司馬談) dated in the first century BC.

52 Scriptures from the 7th century AD report first Buddhist missionaries in China around 200 BC. An establishing of a stable contact via the 'Silk Road' however can not be identified before the first century AD (c.f. Hill 2009).

Confucianism

One of the most famous passages in Chinese philosophy dealing with human emotions is in the chapter *Li Yun* (禮運) of the Book of Rites (*Liji*禮記), one of the books which is attributed to Confucius (*Kong Fuzi* 孔夫子).

何謂人情？喜怒哀懼愛惡欲七者，弗學而能.[53]

> What are the human emotions? Happiness, anger, sadness, fear, love, hate and desire are the seven [emotions], [these emotions] do not have to be learned.

Here the human emotions happiness, anger, sadness, fear, love, hate and desire are mentioned and are described as being 'innate'; one can see a significant similarity to the modern psychological concept of the 'basic emotions' as described in chapter one of this dissertation. This Confucian text also holds the opinion that humans are born and equipped with a specific set of emotions as basic equipment. Additionally, the text *Xunzi* (荀子), attributed to the Confucian philosopher of the same name, provides a very similar statement concerning the 'innateness' of a set of emotions in human:

散名之在人者：生之所以然者謂之性.[...]性之好，惡，喜，怒，哀，樂謂之情.
情然而心為之擇謂之慮.[54]

> What human defines by birth is called his nature. [...] Parts of this nature are liking, hate, happiness, anger, sadness and joy, which are called emotions. If an emotion arises, but the mind chooses different, this is called [rational] thinking.

Xunzi names the option of rational thinking in order to suppress or at least to modify emotionality, but also states that human emotions are inborn. So consequently for Xunzi, human nature is embedded between the conflicting poles of emotion and rational thinking.

Returning to the *Liji*, the chapter *Zhongyong* (中庸) emphasizes the importance of creating an emotional equilibrium, an ideal state which is to be achieved according to Confucian belief. Furthermore, it denotes the important

---

53 Liji禮記, Li Yun 禮運 18.
54 Xunzi荀子, Zhengming 正名 2.

relationship between harmony on an individual, a microcosmic, and on global and macrocosmic levels.

喜怒哀樂之未發, 謂之中 ; 發而皆中節 , 謂之和 ; 中也者 , 天下之大本也 ; 和也者 , 天下之達道也 . 致中和 , 天地位焉 , 萬物育焉 .[55]

> If happiness, anger, sadness and joy are not stirred up, [the mind] is in balance. If [these emotions] are stirred up, but in an appropriate measure, it leads to harmony. Balance is the fundament of everything in the world. Harmony is the way for everybody to proceed. If balance and harmony are established, heaven and earth are in peace and all things are nourished and flourishing.

Although there are no explicit systematic connections between harmony or balance and states of illness and suffering, this excerpt clearly emphasizes the importance of emotional equilibrium. 'Harmony' (*he* 和) here is usually understood as a "dynamic state of creative interchange [and] as the supreme form of value or goodness" (Chen 1991: 251). This relates to a basic feature of Confucian philosophy: to connect the micro- and the macro-levels. For this school of thought, the harmony of the cosmos is rooted in the harmony of the individual and its family. If the individual's self is in a harmonic state, then the family is in harmony as well. If the families are balanced, so is the village. If the villages are in equilibrium, then so are the provinces; and finally, if the provinces are in harmony, this leads to a harmonious country; with harmonious countries, a harmonious cosmos is established (c.f. Yao 2000: 184).[56]

Yao (2000) explains the character *he* 和 as composed of a stylised plant (禾 left part) and a stylised mouth (口 right part) to be a simplified substitute for the older character *he* 龢 which is composed of *he* 禾 on the right side as a hint for its pronunciation and *yue* 龠 on the left. This character *yue* 龠 is derived from an oracle-bone pictograph and shows a panpipe with three holes. The author therefore suggests that in ancient times music and harmony were closely related; that music was seen as essential to develop a good character and that music could not only harmonise human sentiments but also bring order out of social

---

55 Liji 禮記, Zhongyong 中庸 1.
56 The importance of harmony is by no means only a phenomenon of ancient China. For example the Newspaper China Daily, even in its English language version, claims harmony to be the basis for the Olympic Games in 2008: "'One World, One Dream' is simple in expressions, but profound in meaning. It reflects the values of harmony connoted in the concept of 'People's Olympics'" (China Daily, 09.08.2008).

chaos (Yao 2000: 171).[57] Music's modulating effect on emotion played an important role in correctly observing the Confucian ritual (*li* 禮), where music was an integral part of the performance itself (Nylan 2001: 111-112). Hsu estimates that by music "rhythms of sociality" and the "morality of the right way", represented by the song-line as a metaphor for the *dao* (道), could be imparted among the attendants (Hsu 2007: 123).[58]

Also the *Lunyu* (論語), the "Analects of Confucius", deals with emotions. However, emotions are only a sub-item in the broader discussion of the human character, referring to Confucian concepts like 'virtue' (*de* 德), 'benevolence' (*ren* 仁) and 'filial piety' (*xiao* 孝). In the chapter *Xian Wen* (憲問), it is written:

> 克, 伐, 怨, 欲不行焉, 可以為仁矣？子曰：可以為難矣, 仁則吾不知也.[59]
>
> When the love of superiority, boasting, hate, and desire are repressed, this may be deemed perfect virtue. The Master said: This may be regarded as the achievement of what is difficult. But I do not know that it is to be deemed perfect virtue.

As said before, the Confucian concept of harmony is specifically focused on human relationships and social interaction. It does not totally neglect one's individual feelings, but aims to incorporate the appropriate feeling in a certain situation or circumstance, without going into extreme excess of emotional utterances. Additionally, there is an explicit moral dimension in Confucian thought about emotionality. Emotional harmony is closely connected to a more general concept of harmony as a overarching principle which is inseparably related to dif-

---

57   The character 樂 if pronounced le means joy, if pronounced yue means music. Da'an Pan therefore estimates that this similarity "semiotically suggests the positive effects of music on emotional health" (Pan 2003: 253).

58   In the same paragraph Hsu speculates about a connection between ancient China and contemporary Southeast Asia as a larger cultural region, were the role of music respectively the singing of a shaman and the song-line as a metaphor for a moral guide-line are perceived in a similar way (ibid. 123). I think this close connection is questionable. If there are these similarities indeed, it is also likely that different people at different times and in different places used the same metaphorical approach. She herself emphasizes that the medical theories and practices of these temporally and spatially totally different cultural settings "reflect historically contingent cultural specificity" (ibid.).

59   Lunyu (論語) Xian wen (憲問) 1.

ferent spheres like nature, politics, ethics and the everyday life (Yao 2000: 172, c.f. Hagen 2003). Or, as Cheng Chung-Yin explains:

> Right actions and good people induce good feeling, and wrong actions and bad people induce bad feelings which would then lead to an effort to transform the bad into the good, or an effort to cancel the wrong through the exertion of the right, which would normally mean punitive action against the wrong and self-cultivation of the good (Cheng 2001: 85).

Confucianism holds that emotionality is only appropriate in a specific situation within the framework of ritual prescriptions and moral norms and rejects emotions if they are in excess or against the moral order.

Daoism

Daoism suggests that the pristine condition of human was uncontaminated by emotions and therefore it attempts to re-establish this primordial condition (Hendrischke 2001: 106). Daoist philosophy tries to achieve this through different paths. One path deals with reducing and suppressing emotions because this then leads to a more economic consumption of life energy in order to fulfil the main task of Daoist philosophy, i.e. to prolong life or even achieve immortality (c.f. Engelhardt 2000). Another approach is to unmask the postulated absurdity of emotional experience in the social context and to understand that emotional response and involvement misdirects humans (Hendrischke 2001: 106). However, this does not mean that Daoist philosophy absolutely rejects emotions. It clearly rejects emotions in the Confucian way, i.e. emotionality is appropriate only in certain situations and regulated according to rites and rules. Daoist philosophy, on the contrary, claims that there is a natural, pristine condition of human existence which should be achieved. In this pristine state, emotional experience is possible without the influence of principles, social rules and restrictions.[60]

---

60 There seems to be a contradiction or at least an ambiguity in Daoist thought and terminology about emotions. From this point of view, emotions are socially constructed and therefore should be suppressed in order to achieve a pristine state of "calmness and nihility" (Liu 2011:121). In this state, a 'genuine' emotional experience should be possible. Some authors like Liu Qingping (2011) try to clarify this ambiguity by differenti-

Thus, the *Guanzi* (管子)[61], an encyclopaedic compilation of early Chinese philosophical texts containing Legalist and Daoist thoughts, outlines in the treatise *Xinshu* (心術), which according to Hendrischke (2001: 108) is safe to be thought of containing mainly Daoist ideas:

凡民之生也，必以正平，所以失之者，必以喜樂哀怒。[62]

Everyone's nature is to be unadulterated and even, but this will be lost through happiness, joy, sadness and anger.

This passage emphasizes the Daoist notion of an original human state uncontaminated by emotions. Consequently, in another chapter of the same book the author pleas for the overcoming of emotionality. This avoidance of emotional involvement then should lead to harmony:

能去憂樂喜怒欲利，心乃反濟。彼心之情，利安以寧，勿煩勿亂，和乃自成 [63]

If one gets rid of sorrow, joy, happiness, anger and of desiring profits, the heart will be relieved again. The sentiment of the heart will be in serenity, avoiding confusion and chaos, harmony will prevail.

Hence, the emerging of emotions and their culturally shaped significance is perceived to be opposed to a natural, pristine state of harmony. In the Daoist clascial treatise *Zhuangzi* (莊子)[64], attributed to a philosopher of the same name, one

---

      ating between 'emotions' and 'feeling'. In this context, the term emotions describes the socially constructed emotions which Daoism wants to overcome, while the term feeling means the pristine, natural emotional experience which Daoism wants to achieve.
61   This text is usually dated to the first century BC, acknowledging that its roots may be in the 4th century BC.
62   Guanzi管子, Xin Shu II心術下 6.
63   Guanzi管子, Nei Ye內業 1.
64   The book Zhuangzi is commonly regarded as a composition of different texts. Whether the authorship of 4th century philosopher Zhuangzi is verifiable, remains unclear. The basis for later editions of the text is a recension of the 3rd century AD.

finds an interesting discussion between the philosopher Zhuangzi and one of his disciples who doubts this general opinion:[65]

> 惠子謂莊子曰: '人故無情乎?' 莊子曰 : '然.' 惠子曰 : '人而無情, 何以謂之人?' 莊子曰 : '道與之貌, 天與之形, 惡得不謂之人?' 惠子曰 : '既謂之人, 惡得無情?' 莊子曰 : '是非吾所謂情也. 吾所謂無情者, 言人之不以好惡內傷其身, 常因自然而不益生也.'[66]

> Huizi asked Zhuangzi: 'Can human be without emotions?' Zhuangzi answered: 'Of course.' Huizi said: 'A human without emotions, how can you call him human?' Zhuangzi answered: 'The Dao gives him attitude; Heaven gives him bodily form, why should I not call him human?' Huizi said, 'But what you call human, how can he be without emotions?' Zhuangzi answered: '[What you mean by emotions,] Is not what I mean by emotions. What I mean by saying without emotion is, that this human does not through love and hate internally harm his body, but keeps his regular natural [pristine condition] without adding anything to life.'

In a second passage of the same book, *Zhuangzi* again explains not to externalize feelings according to appropriate behaviour in a Confucian sense, but be 'natural' in order to become a 'true' or 'genuine' (*zhen* 真) human:

> 真者, 精誠之至也。不精不誠, 不能動人。故強哭者雖悲不哀, 強怒者雖嚴不威, 強親者雖笑不和。真悲無聲而哀, 真怒未發而威, 真親未笑而和。[...]禮者, 世俗之所為也; 真者, 所以受於天也, 自然不可易也.[67]

> *Zhen* means purity and sincerity in the highest degree. Without purity and sincerity, one can not move [other] people. Hence strong crying, however sad, shows no [real] grief. Strong anger, however stern, will not terrify [anyone]. Strong affection, however smiley, does not lead to harmony. True sadness makes no noise yet [shows] grief, true anger without being expressed will be terrifying, true affection without smiling will lead to harmony. [...] The rites have been made for the ordinary people; the true human has received [trueness] from heaven, [which is therefore] indeed natural and unchangeable.

---

65 There is a discussion about the character qing 情 used in this paragraph, which means 'emotion' or 'feeling', but can also be translated as 'essential' (Hendrischke 2001: 112). For a deeper insight see Hansen 1995.
66 Zhuangzi 莊子, De Chong Fu 德充符 6.
67 Zhuangzi 莊子, Yu Fu 漁父 5.

As one can see, for Zhuangzi the way to proceed is not as "vulgar learning such as Confucian schools" (Xiang 2008: 504) recommends, but to return to the original and natural existence, in which "human nature as pure spontaneity of heaven" only cared to satisfy some basic needs like ingestion and rest and in which emotions were reactions to "external phenomena [...] spontaneously expressed in manifestations of happiness and sorrow" (Santangelo 1999: 200). Wolfgang Bauer (1971: 64) calls this existence "pre-human" (*vormenschlich*). In this condition, one can exist "free from all human sorrows" (*allen menschlichen Sorgen enthoben*) and acts spontaneously and "unconscious", meaning that one is unconscious and unadulterated of social and restriction bounds.

As for the Daoists, the universe in its origin is believed to be empty, silent, tranquil and non-active; the way to achieve this original state again is to non-act (Santangelo 1999: 200).

Very similar to the other classical Daoist texts quoted above, the *Huainanzi* (淮南子), a text written in the earlier Han-Dynasty (202 BC – 6 AD), also deals with emotions and emphasizes their influence on human the body. It characterises emotions as deeply disturbing and stirring. The following paragraph shows the connection between emotional experience and bodily reaction:

人之性有侵犯則怒，怒則血充，血充則氣激，氣激則發怒，發怒則有所釋憾矣。[68]

It is part of human nature that if something invades and violates [a human being], this leads to anger, anger leads to a replenishment of blood, replenishment of blood leads to arousing *qi*, aroused *qi* leads to an emission of anger, emission of anger leads to a release of one's dissatisfaction.

This chain of cause-and-effect which leads to an emission of anger characterises the emotion of anger not only as connected to the bodily experience of disturbing *qi*, but also to have the inherit quality of emission, which consequently provokes its manifestation to the outside. This chain reaction is what Daoism tries to avoid; if one wants to overcome the existence of an ordinary human in order to become a sage, one has to overcome the dependencies of human life and to free oneself from the burden of emotions (Vankeerberghen 1995: 528-529).

---

68   Huainanzi淮南子, Benjing Xun本經訓 5.

Similar Aim, Different Approaches

Whereas Confucianism claims that people should engage in political life according to moral principles like filial piety and benevolence and thus take action, Daoism wants people to 'act through non-acting' (*wu wei* 無為). Involvement with the world and emotional experience are seen as harmful for the body; therefore the natural, primordial condition should be achieved. Daoism in general rejects the value of wisdom, desire or benevolence in the Confucian sense not so much because it is 'emotionless', but because of the psychological factors that encourages people to act in order to achieve these values. These psychological factors detain human in social institutions such as "business affairs, social activities and personal matters" and prevent them from aspiring to "calmness and nihility" (Wang 1991: 28-29). For the Daoist, "civilization and society could not be helpful in the emotional field, but they worsen man's situation and damage human life" (Santangelo 1999: 206). Alternatively, Daoism holds that there is a spontaneous way of feeling, an initial emotional impulse which is more 'genuine'. For Laozi (老子), the legendary philosopher who is believed to be the founder of Daoism, "affectionate love is not an artificial emotion like the human love advocated by Confucianism, but a natural feeling by which people can achieve a spontaneous unity with heaven" (Liu 2011: 121). What Liu calls "affectionate love" here is the special kind of 'feeling' of people who reached the Daoist's goal of achieving primordial condition of life again. Consequently, the public exhibition of strong emotional affection, what Liu calls "human love", is considered to be insincere because it infringes the Daoist's aim to be 'true' or 'genuine' (*zhen* 真).

By now we have a twofold condemnation of strong emotional affection represented in the two main philosophical schools in China: Confucianism denotes strong emotionality to be against the moral order and against the prescriptions of the ritual. It only permits a specific amount of emotionality in accordance to specific situations. Daoism rejects emotions by calling them artificial and insincere. From this point of view, emotionality is a social construct which has to be replaced by the natural flow of 'acting through non-acting' (*wu wei* 無為).

These philosophical attitudes were always considered to be especially relevant for Chinese medicine. For example, one of the most famous ancient books on Chinese medicine, the *Huangdi neijing* (黃帝內經 'Yellow Emperor's Classic on Internal Medicine'), which will be dealt with in the subsequent chapter, for a long period of time was preserved in a Daoist Canon compiled between 1445 and 1447 (Engelfried 2000: 254 & 248). The close connection between philosophy and medicine also comes to light in statements like that of the Song-Dynasty (960-1279) statesmen Fan Zhongyan (范仲淹) from whom is recorded that "if one cannot become a minister one should become a doctor". Confucianism and Daoism, beside other philosophical schools, were perceived as especially relevant for medicine, as Ming-Dynasty (1368-1644) physician Sun Yikui (孫一奎) states in his medical work called "The Dark Pearl of the Red Water" (*chishui xuan zhu* 赤水玄珠)[69]:

> The Confucians' investigation of principles and exhaustion of nature to reach at destiny, should serve as the standard against which to gauge. On the other hand, from the Taoists' cultivating nature and destiny together, [...] the principles of the way may also be gleaned. Therefore I have drawn on both traditions in order that they may serve as wings (Sun Yikui, cited in Engelfriet 2000: 253).

Classical Medical Texts and the Impact of Emotions

As already mentioned, there is a vast amount of medical literature preserved; among them the most famous writings *Huangdi neijing* (黃帝內經 'Yellow Emperor's Classic on Internal Medicine' (HDNJ)) and the *Nanjing* (難經 'Classic on Difficult Questions' (NJ)), which deal with a more generalized view on inner medicine. Furthermore, there are also many writings on pharmacology (for example the *Bencao gangmu* 本草綱目 'Compendium of Materia Medica' or the *Shennong bencao jing* 神農本草經 'Shennong's Classic on Materia Media') and on special illnesses (for example *Shanghang lun* 傷寒論 'Treatise on Cold Damage Disorder'). In order to work out the connection between emotions and illness represented in these particular texts, I shall now analyze some chosen passages of the HDNJ, the NJ and some other classical texts on Chinese medicine.

69　Engelfried explains that the title is an allusion to the 12th chapter of the Zhuangzi, in which the Yellow Emperor is looking for his 'Dark Pearl' which he lost while ascending the Mount Kunlun. Engelfried furthermore shows that Sun not only took a Daoist view, but also reflects Neo-Confucian and Buddhist perspectives (Engelfried 2000: 249, 251).

The Huangdi neijing

The HDNJ is commonly assigned to the mythological Yellow Emperor who is believed to have ruled China 4500 years ago and invented several cultural techniques like the Chinese writing system; he is also believed to be the founder of Chinese medicine. For the Chinese, this book marks the beginning of Chinese medicine and at present, according to *zhongyi*-doctors, the HDNJ is a standard reference and specific passages are usually and regularily cited.[70] Today, scholars assume that the text is a collection of different earlier writings from a Daoist as well as from a Confucian background and that it was compiled during the 3rd or 2nd century BC (Jewell 1990: 229).[71]

In the HDNJ there are several passages which outline the connection between emotions and illness. The following paragraph enumerates the causes of illness:

> 黃帝問于歧伯曰：夫百病之始生也，皆生於風雨寒暑，清濕喜怒，喜怒不節則傷藏，風雨則傷上，清濕則傷下.[72]

> The Yellow Emperor inquired Qi Bo saying: The hundred [meaning: all] illnesses have their origin in wind, rain, cold, heat, coolness, dampness, joy and anger, joy and anger injure the *zang* [*zang*-Organs, the depots][73], wind and rain injure the upper [body parts], coolness and dampness injure the lower [body parts].

70　Matten (2009: 55-61) explains that the Yellow Emperor had to act in different roles in Chinese History and his role changed from being an Emperor and founder of a Chinese kingdom to being the progenitor of the Han and later of the multiethnic Chinese nation (Zhongguo minzu 中国民族) and a culture hero. Matten strikingly comments that „the Yellow Emperor somehow is everything, but not always at the same time" (61). Dirlik (1996b, c.f. Pan 1990) exposes clearly that the myth of the Yellow Emperor since the end of the Mao era is gaining more and more importance and therefore induces a kind of "revival" of the Yellow Emperor "as the historical ancestor of the Chinese people, whose ancestry still binds together Chinese around the world" (Dirlik 1996b: 250). C.f. Akahori (1989: 19), who denotes that the HDNJ is a standard reference in contemporary Japanese Medicine, too.

71　C.f. Unschuld (1995: 30) who assumes that the core of the HDNJ is dated from the 2nd century BC and that its oldest parts which deal with illnesses caused by wind are even older.

72　Huangdi neijing黃帝內經, Lingshu 靈樞, Baibing shisheng 百病始生 1.

73　See chapter 1.

In addition to climatic factors, joy and anger as prototypes of human emotions[74] demarking extreme emotional conditions of either wellbeing or distress are named as causing illnesses. This differentiation of illness instigators reflects the divide of pathogenic factors into outer causes (i.e. climatic factors) and inner causes (i.e. emotions), a dichotomy which is prevalent in Chinese medical theory.[75] The attribution of emotions to certain organs already is implied, as emotions are said to injure the *zang* organs; however, there is no clear relation of certain emotions to specific organs, as it is worked out in later medical texts.

Regarding the well-known equation of emotional equilibrium and moderation on the one hand and health respectively a better and more worriless life on the other hand one finds in the HDNJ following passage:

是以志閑而少欲，心安而不懼.[76]

Thus if emotions are constraint, there are fewer desires, if the heart is in peace, there is no fear anymore.

The following quote from the Chapter *Yinyang yinxian dalun* (陰陽應象大論) of the HDNJ states that emotions are as 'natural' as the different seasons. But as humans have to live with the seasons and have to cope with their climatic extremes, which act on the body but also may cause bad harvests, one can conclude that, although emotions are 'natural', one has to endure the consequences of being excessively emotional.

天有四時五行，以生長收藏，以生寒暑燥濕風。人有五藏，化五氣，以生喜怒悲憂恐。故喜怒傷氣，寒暑傷形。暴怒傷陰，暴喜傷陽。厥氣上行，滿脈去形。喜怒不節，寒暑過度，生乃不固.[77]

In the world there are four seasons and five phases, [the first] one brings birth, growing, harvest and storing, [the second] one brings cold, heat, drought, dampness and wind. Human has five *zang* [*zang*-Organs, the depots] that convert five [types of] *qi*, bringing joy, anger, sadness, sorrow and fear. Hence joy and anger injure *qi*, cold

---

74　For a detailed discussion of the emotion terms used in the HDNJ I refer to Messner 2006.
75　See chapter 1.
76　Huangdi neijing 黃帝內經, Suwen 素問, Shanggu tian zhen lun 上古天真論 2.
77　Huangdi neijing 黃帝內經, Suwen 素問, Yinyang yinxiang dalun 陰陽應象大論 6.

and heat injure the form [the body]. Excessive anger injures the *yin*, excessive joy injures the *yang*. The *qi* flows upwards [in the body], the vessels are filled and [their contents] leave the body. If joy and anger are not restraint, if cold and heat break through certain limits, then life is not solid.

These consequences are denoted as injuring the *qi*, throwing out of balance the ratio of *yin* and of *yang* and thus finally disturbing the solid foundation of life. Additionally, this passage is a particular elaboration and reinforcement of the first cited paragraph of the HDNJ. It again shows the differentiation into external causes, cold and heat, which inflicts 'outer' human parts, the form (*xing* 形) or the "physical appearance" (Messner 2006: 42), and the internal causes, joy and anger, which affect with 'inner' parts of humans, the *qi* (氣).

In conclusion, one might say that the HDNJ describes the necessity of "moderating the emotional processes" and denotes the autonomy from "worldly desires as the most beneficial state of being for health and longevity" (Messer 2006: 59).

The Nanjing

The *Nanjing* (難經), or 'Classic of Difficult Issues', very likely compiled during the 1st and 2nd century AD, was one of the most authoritative texts in Chinese Medicine until the end of the first millennium. It was succeeded and in some cases displaced by the earlier HDNJ, which gained more and more importance and influence and hence downgraded the NJ in the opinion of scholars and doctors to an interesting, but limited annotation of the HDNJ. Nevertheless, Unschuld states that the NJ should still be "regarded as a significant and innovative work" (Unschuld 1986: 3).

The first chapter of the NJ, the *Jing mei zhenhou* (經脈診候), makes statements about the relationship between emotions and illnesses:

然：假令得肝脈，其外證：善潔，面青，善怒；其內證：齊左有動氣，按之牢若痛．[...] 假令得心脈，其外證：面赤，口乾，喜笑；其內證：齊上有動氣，按之牢若痛．[...]假令得脾脈，其外證：面黃，善噫，善思，善味；其內證：當齊有動氣，按之牢若痛[...]假令得肺脈，其外證：面白，善嚏，悲愁不樂，

欲哭；其內證：齊右有動氣，按之牢若痛．[...]假令得腎脈，其外證：面黑，喜恐欠；其內證：齊下有動氣，按之牢若痛．⁷⁸

Actually it is like this: If there is a disturbance in a vessel associated to the liver, its external evidences are increased cleanliness, a greenish face and increased [tendency to become] angry; its internal evidence is the movement of *qi* inside [the body] on the left side of the navel [causing] firm and painful sensation if pressed. [...] If there is a disturbance in a vessel associated to the heart, its external evidences are a reddish face, a dry mouth and increased [tendency to] laugh; its internal evidence is the movement of *qi* inside [the body] on the upper side of the navel [causing] firm and painful sensation if pressed. [...] If there is a disturbance in a vessel associated to the spleen, its external evidences are a yellowish face, a tendency to belch and to ponder and to [enjoy] tasty [food]; its internal evidence is the movement of *qi* inside [the body] on the spot of the navel [causing] firm and painful sensation if pressed. [...] If there is a disturbance in a vessel associated to the lungs, its external evidences are a pale face, a tendency to sneeze and [a tendency to feel] sorrow and anxiety without joy and a longing to cry; its internal evidence is the movement of *qi* inside [the body] on the right side of the navel [causing] firm and painful sensation if pressed. [...]If there is a disturbance in a vessel associated to the kidney, its external evidences are a blackish face, a tendency to be fearful and to yawn; its external evidence is the movement of *qi* to the lower side of the navel [causing] firm and painful sensation if pressed.

In this quoted initial chapter of the NJ, the connection between emotions and illnesses is explained by naming first the locus of disturbance and then denotes certain emotional states as symptoms, to use a biomedical term here, in order to describe the disturbance and to explain it. This is not the usual way of listing the relationship between emotions and illness in classical Chinese texts. As demonstrated above, usually the texts start with the naming of emotions and then attribute specific organs. Hence, according to the concept of the Five Phases and the theory of systematic correspondence[79], this reversed connection is plausible. However, in later chapters of the NJ, one can find the more usual relationship between emotions and illnesses, i.e. emotions not as symptoms but as causes of certain disease:

然：經言憂愁思慮則傷心；形寒飲冷則傷肺；恚怒氣逆，上而不下則傷肝；飲食勞倦則傷脾；久坐濕地，強力入水則傷腎．⁸⁰

---

78 Nanjing 難經, Jing mei zhenhou 經脈診候 17.
79 See chapter 1.
80 Nanjing 難經, Xiushi xie zheng 虛實邪正 2.

Actually it is like this: the classic [book][81] says that grief, anxiety, pondering and worry injure the heart; a cold body and cold drinks injure the lungs; rage and anger [leads to] misbehaving *qi* moving upward instead of moving downward [and by this] injure the liver. [Extensive] eating and drinking and exhausting labour injure the spleen; sitting in a moist surrounding, overexerting ones strength and going into water injures the kidneys.

Although according to the concept of the Five Phases, theoretically every organ has a corresponding emotion; it the quote above, the heart and the liver are likely to be affected (in the true sense of the word). There is some evidence in commentaries to this specific passage of the NJ that in fact more emotions are included in this paragraph, but hidden in metaphorical formulations. According to a 3rd century commentary by the author Lü Kuang (呂曠), this specific phrase 'sitting in a moist surrounding' (*zuo shidi* 坐濕地) should be read as "to meet with grief and mourning", but nevertheless the main motive of this cited passage of the NJ in all probability is what the 14th century doctor Hua Shou (滑 壽) summarized in his commentary on this paragraph:

> Of course, man cannot get along without grief, thoughts, rage, food and drink, movement and exertion. If the development [of these states] remains in a medium range, how could they result in injuries?! However, in case of excess, harm to man is inevitable (*Hua Shou* and *Lü Kuang*, both cited in Unschuld 1986: 462-463).

So here once again one finds the concept of 'inborn' emotions as a common feature of human existence, but the fear of excess and the necessity of achieving harmony in one's emotional life in order to avoid illness is described as an omnipresent threat in all treatises.

Miscellaneous Classical Medical Texts

Alongside these two texts, the HDNJ that is still cited in modern China as a standard reference text for *zhongyi*-doctors, and the NJ, which according to Unschuld "provoked the largest numbers of commentaries through the subsequent

---

81 For the discussion whether the formula ‚the classic book says' is a reference to the HDNJ or to other scriptures maybe of legendary origin, see Unschuld 1986: 31-34.

centuries" (Unschuld: 1985: 85) there are several other classical Chinese texts on medical issues which outline the direct link between emotions and illness.

In the early 7th century, Chao Yuanfang (巢元方) wrote the book *Zhu bing yuan hou lun* (諸病源侯論) which should become the first book in Chinese medicine dealing exclusively with aetiology and enumerates a larger number of different illnesses and their origins (Kovacs & Unschuld 1998: 29). It also provides more precise information about the pathogenic potential of emotions:

> "The hundred illnesses have their origin in the influences. Anger causes the influences to rise [in the body]. Joy slows [the flow] of influences. Fear causes the influences to descend [in the body]. Vexation reduces the influences. [...] Grief brings the influences into confusion. [...] Anger reverses the normal flow of the influences. In severe cases the victims cough up blood and food, i.e., the influences ascend. Joy occasions harmony [among the influences]. The constructive and defensive influences flow unobstructed, bestowing their benefits throughout the entire body. This, in turn, diminishes the flow of the [remaining] influences. Vexation causes the large vessel that flow from the heart to contract, and the lobes of the lung begin to rise. This blocks the conduits flowing through the upper burner, preventing dispersal of the constructive and defensive influences and causing heat-influences to accumulate within [the body]. The influences begin to diminish. Fear reduces the essence. A reduction of essence causes the upper burner to close. When this occurs, the influences are forced to reverse their flow, causing swelling in the lower burner and the influences are unable to proceed. [...] When someone grieves, the senses have no place to rest, the spirit has no place to withdraw to, and the mind is confused. As a result, the influences fall into disarray" (*Zhu bing yuan hou lun* (諸病源侯論), in: Unschuld 1985: 299).

This text emphasises the impact of emotions on *qi* (which Unschuld translates as "influence"), whereby anger leads to rising *qi* and fear causes *qi* to descend, joy causes a slowing of *qi*, and grief leads to the confusion of *qi*. Thus, certain emotions, when in excess, influence the state and thus feature of *qi*; in accordance with the Five Phases, it leads to the maladjustment of the whole person.

The treatise *San yin ji yi bingzheng fang lun* (三因極一病證方論) written in the early 12th century by a doctor named Chen Yan (陳言) enumerates the Seven Emotions joy, anger, mourning, excessive thought, grief, fear and fright and calls them 'natural', but harmful in excess:

七請者喜怒憂思悲恐驚是也若將護得宜怡然安泰役冒非理百病生焉. [...] 然六淫天之常氣冒之則先自經絡流入內合於藏府為外所因七請人之常性動之則先自藏府鬱發外形於肢體為內所因.

The seven emotions are joy and anger, mourning and thought, grief, fear and fright. If one, in his effort to preserve (his health), pursues a suitable (way of life, he will, as a result,) be happy and remain free from any disturbance. If, (however, one leads a) risky (life that) is not in accordance with the principles (of nature), all possible illnesses may emerge as a consequence. [...] However, the six essences are ordinary influence from heaven. If one fails to care about (their assimilation in correct proportions), they will flow into (the body) starting from the (major) conduits and network (conduits, and, then,) unite internally in the viscera and bowels. They are causes (of illnesses) that have come from outside. The seven emotions are ordinary (attributes of) human nature. If one excites them, they will be set free first in the viscera and bowels, and (then) they will take shape in (the appearance of man's) limbs and body.[82]

According to this text and as a general principle of Chinese medicine, to neglect harmony leads to "all possible illnesses" (*bai bing* 百病). This principle can also be detected in text *Piwei lun* (脾胃論) written by Li Gao (李杲) in 1249. Here, the author explains the importance of harmony. *Yin* and *yang* should be balanced according to the influence of external factors like the seasons, consumption, and emotionality, which are identified as weakening.

合於四時五臟陰陽揆度以為常也.若飲食失節寒溫不適則脾胃乃傷.喜怒憂恐損源氣.既脾胃氣衰元氣不足而心火獨盛.

If the *yin* and *yang* (influences) in the five viscera (increase and decrease) in accordance with the (course of the) four seasons, this is considered to be normal. If however one drinks and eats without any restraints, and if (one's consumption of drinks and food) fails to correspond to the cold or warmth (of the four seasons), this will cause harm to both spleen and stomach. (Also, excessive) joy and anger, as well as (excessive) mourning and fear injure one's original influences. If the influences of the spleen and of the stomach are weakened, and if not enough original influences are present, a fire will flare up uncontrolled in the heart.[83]

---

82 San yin ji yi bingzheng fang lun (三因極一病證方論), Text and translation in: Unschuld 1988: 100.
83 Piwei lun (脾胃論), Text and translation in: Unschuld 1988: 138.

The later *Yixue yuan liu lun* (醫學源流論), written in 1757 by Xu Dachun (徐大椿), still knows the pathological quality of emotions and denotes that the Seven Emotions are internal causes of illnesses:

七情所病謂之內傷 [...] 內傷由於神志.

Illnesses related to the seven emotions are called „harm from inside". [...] Harm from inside originates from one's spirit and mind.[84]

The several above cited medical texts show that emotionality was considered to be 'normal' and 'natural' by scholars and physicians; however, they were also viewed as a perpetual danger to one's health. This seems to be a Confucian concept of emotions rather than a Daoist one and it implicates the moral commandment of regulating emotions and showing (and feeling one might say) suitable and appropriate feelings. Chao (2009) demonstrates that Confucian philosophy in particular, has influenced medical theory at least since the early 10th century. The author shows that mainly Confucian physicians have been in scholarly positions and have been responsible for most of the written sources assessable today whereas Daoist physicians mainly operated as folk healers without producing a comprehensive textual corpus (Chao 2009: 25-52). However, describing classical Chinese medical texts, Hsu (2007) claims that Chinese medicine "appealed to the responsibility of the self for the self and advocated regularity in food intake and drinking, [...] feelings and emotions" and by this it was a "medicine of moderation" (Hsu 2007: 118). In the following paragraph I analyse recently published medical textbooks. With these modern books I shall demonstrate that Chinese medicine not only was, but still is a "medicine of moderation" where emotions are concerned.

---

84   Yixue yuan liu lun (醫學源流論), text and translation in: Unschuld 1990: 106-107. He translates zhi 志 here as 'mind', but it has a broader meaning and is commonly also translated as 'emotion'. Even if in this context the translation 'mind' is more appropriate, the ambiguity of this term has to be recognized.

4. Emotions and Health in Modern Medical Textbooks

The classical texts of Chinese philosophy and medicine and their discussion concerning emotionality and illness lay the foundation for Chinese medicine's modern interpretation and consideration of the pathological risk of being emotional. I present a selective number of recently published textbooks on Chinese medicine and intend to demonstrate that today the connections of emotions and illness are still perceived as deep and influential despite the few differences in the selected textbooks when it comes to therapeutic principles and treatment options.

The starting point and beginning of a "50-year history of textbooks" conceptually forming Chinese medicine (Hsu 2008: 467) doubtlessly is the *Zhongyixue gailun* (中医学概论 'Introduction to Chinese Medicine'), which was published in its first edition in 1958. This book, as quoted in Ots (1999), presents an argument similar to the classical texts, connecting the health risks of emotionality mainly to their excess:

> „Die Stimmungslage und der Zustand des Denkens haben auf die Entstehung und die Entwicklung von Krankheiten großen Einfluss. Die chinesische Medizin legt größten Wert auf die Veränderung der Stimmung und ihre Beziehung zur Krankheit, die sich phänomenologisch durch die sieben Emotionen äußern. [...]Die sieben Emotionen repräsentieren den durch jedwede äußeren Reize konstituierten psychischen Zustand des Menschen. Unter normalen äußeren Bedingungen und bei normaler physiologischer Aktivität induzieren die sieben Emotionen keinerlei Krankheit. Sollten die Reize aber zu stark oder langandauernd sein, oder wenn der Mensch sie nicht korrekt verarbeiten kann, kommt es zu drastischen emotionalen Veränderungen und mithin zu Krankheit. [...] Obwohl die von den sieben Emotionen induzierten Erkrankungen sich auf alle fünf *zang*-Organe beziehen können, zeigt die klinische Praxis dennoch, dass die von den sieben Emotionen am stärksten betroffenen Organe das Herz, die Leber und die Milz sind. (*Zhongyixue gailun*, cited in: Ots 1999: 62).[85]

---

85 The mood and the condition of thinking are important fort he origin and the developement of illnesses. Chinese medicine emphasizes the change of mood and its connections to illnesses, which phenomenological are represented in the Seven Emotions. These Seven Emotions represent the psychic condition of human beings, excited through outer irritations. Under normal outer conditions and normal physiological activity, these Sev-

While the book states that emotions and the state of mind ('*Zustand des Denkens*') are important factors concerning the causation and the progression of illnesses and that especially excessive or continuous emotional stimulation is a precursor to illness, it explains that although theoretically all *zang*-organs could be afflicted, the most endangered organs are the heart, the liver and the spleen. As I explain in the upcoming chapter, the special role of these organs, at least the liver and the heart, in terms of the possibility of emotional influence are present in my informant's views as well.

Zhongyi Neikexue (2002)

The *Zhongyi Neikexue* (中医内科学, "Internal Traditional Chinese Medicine"), published in 2002 by the universities of Chinese Medicine in Shanghai and Nanjing evidently denotes the interdependence between emotions and organs when it states that

情志变化可以影响内脏功能，内脏的病变也可以引起情志活动的异常 (p. 12).

Emotional disorders can influence the functions of internal organs, while dysfunctions of internal organs can lead to the disturbance of emotions.

Throughout the book emotions are categorized as inner causes (*nei yin* 内因) or inner injuries (*nei shang* 内伤) and are described as causing different illnesses like depression (*yiyuzheng* 抑郁症), mania (*kuangzheng* 癫狂), wind stroke (*zhongfeng* 中风), vertigo (*xuanyun* 眩晕) or illnesses of the thyroid gland (*yingbing* 瘿病) (ibid.: 3-4). The enumeration of possible pathongenic emotions is wide ranging, starting with more general formulations like "the seven emotions" (*qi qing* 七情) or "emotional imbalance" (*qingzhi shitiao* 情志失调) to more detailed descriptions like "enormous fright and fear" (*da jing da kong* 大惊大恐) or

---

en Emotions induce no illnesses. However, when the irritations are to strong or to long in duration, or if the human being can not process it appropriately, this leads to drastic emotional variations and thus to illnesses. [...] Although the illnesses induced by the Seven Emotions can have reference to all of the five zang-Organs, clinical practice show that the most strongly affected organs by the Seven Emotions are the heart, the liver and the spleen (my translation).

"depression and anger" (*youyu naonu*忧郁恼怒) to a whole list expounding upon "anger, fright, grief, joy and excessive thinking" (*naonu jingkong bei xi silü* 恼怒惊恐悲喜思虑) (ibid.: 83, 95, 116, 210, 125).

Although emotions are identified as pathogenic agents as shown above, they are not named in the chapter "On Therapeutic Principles and Healing Methods in Chinese Internal Medicine" ("中医内科学疾病的治疗原则和常用治法") (ibid. 17-27). The routine treatment referring to the therapeutic principles of "treating a disease contrary to its nature" ("正治也称逆治") means that, for example, a cold syndrome has to be treated by applying drugs of warm nature, whereas a heat syndrome has to be treated by applying drugs of cold nature. The treatment contrary to the routine referring to the principles of "treating a disease according to its nature" ("反治也称从治") demands that cold syndromes should be treated with cold drugs and heat syndromes with warm drugs, as in this specific cases the true origin of the disease (the cold syndrome is indeed a heat syndrome, the heat syndrome is indeed a cold syndrome) is hidden (ibid. 17-18). Both of these therapeutic principles neglect the possibility of adjusting emotions by inducing 'counter-emotions'. Heat and cold as well as deficiency and excess of *yin* and *yang* or *qi* are the main factors to identify and treat diseases. So for the *Zhongyi Neikexue*, emotions are 'somehow' connected to disease and are identified as possible pathogen agents for several specific diseases like the ones listed above; but when it comes to therapeutic principles and treatment, they are more or less neglected. Emotion induced illnesses are treated solely by 'somatic'[86] adjustments. This is a first hint to 'somatization', which I further discuss in the next chapter.

Zhongyi jichu lilun

The *Zhongyi jichu lilun* (中医基础理论 Basic Theory of Traditional Chinese Medicine) published by Liu Yanchi and Liu Zhanwen in 1998 approaches the topic more systematically in devoting a special chapter to the connections between emotions and illness. It names the emotions joy, anger, grief, pensiveness,

---

[86] As shown in Chapter 1, the differentiation between 'soma' and 'psyche' is a phenomenon of western philosophy and psychology, not an Asian one. Nevertheless I use the terms 'soma' and 'psyche' in this chapter, signalized with apostrophe. I do not mean to impose the Cartesian Dualism on Chinese medicine, but I simply show that treatment options, 'biomedically' spoken, refer to 'material', 'soma'-related measures like herbal drugs, or to 'immaterial', 'psyche'-related measures like counselling etc.

worry, fear and fright (*xi* 喜, *nu* 怒, *you* 忧, *si* 思, *bei* 悲, *kong* 恐, *jing* 惊) and states that "normally these emotions can not induce illnesses" ("一般不会使人致病") (p. 373). But if human's emotionality exceeds 'normality', if emotions are stimulated suddenly, very strongly or for a prolonged period of time, they can "disturb the *qi*, influence *yin* and *yang*, blood and the *zangfu*-organs and by this, illnesses can occur" ("[…] 使人体气机紊乱, 脏腑阴阳气血失调, 才会导致疾病的发生") (ibid. 374).

In the paragraphs dealing with the pathological quality of emotions, this book very often cites the *Huangdi neijing* and uses this text as an authority reference. For example it cites two chapters of the HDNJ and contrasts them in order to make the point that although it is said that emotions are connected to and injure certain organs, ("anger injures the liver, joy injures the heart, pensiveness injures the spleen, worry injures the lung, fear injures the kidney" – "怒伤肝, 喜伤心, 思伤脾, 忧伤肺, 恐伤肾") they can also affect other body parts ("the heart is the prince of the five *zang*-organs and the six fu-organs; worry, fright, anger and grief make the heart shake, which makes the five *zang*-organs and the six *fu*-organs shake accordingly" – "心者, 五脏六腑之主也, 故悲惊愁忧则动, 心动则五脏六腑皆摇") (ibid. 374).

The *Zhongyi jichu lilun* furthermore emphasizes that strong emotionality not only may disturb the *qi* or the *yin* and *yang* balance and thereby cause illnesses, but remarks that emotional instability and imbalance may lead to increasing afflictions or to an exacerbation of the general condition ("情志异常波动, 可使病情加重, 或迅速恶化") (ibid. 375).

In contrast to the *Zhongyi neikexue* (2002), where the emotions are named as pathogenic agents, but actually play no important role in concrete illness causations, the *Zhongyi jichu lilun* accentuates the pathogenic potential of emotions more detailed.

Zhongyi neikexue (2007)

The textbook *Zhongyi neikexue* (中医内科学 Internal Traditional Chinese Medicine), edited by Wang Xinyue (王新月, 2007a), also lists the Seven Emotions joy, anger, grief, pensiveness, worry, fear and fright (*xi* 喜, *nu* 怒, *you* 忧, *si* 思, *bei* 悲, *kong* 恐, *jing* 惊) as potentially pathogenic and likewise points out that excess or extreme changes of emotional experience are especially dangerous for the individual health (p. 8). But despite these more general statements, it elaborately shows the connections of emotionality, organs and illnesses. The heart, for example, is seen as being the centre of emotional and thinking activities ("[心] 为情志思维活动之中枢") (ibid. 10). Therefore it is threatened by extensive thinking and contemplation, which leads to stagnation of *qi* and blood causing an "excess syndrome of the heart" (" 心之实证") (see Fig. 5).

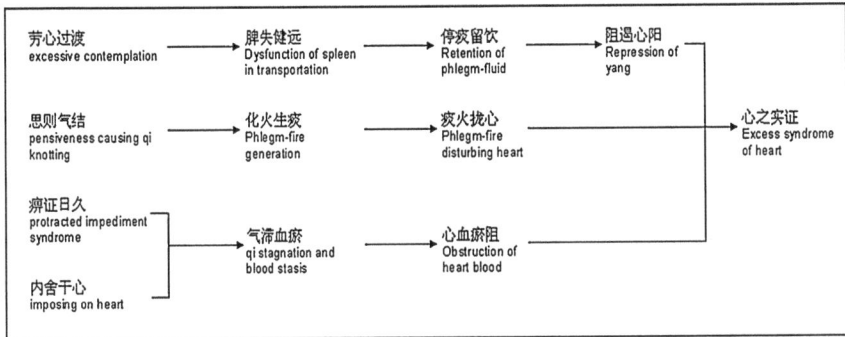

Fig. 5: *Pathogenesis of Heart Disease (segment) (Wang 2007a: 10).*

According to the *Zhongyi neikexue* as well as other medical textbooks, not only the heart but also the liver is very likely to be affected by emotional excess. This organ is said to be the regulator of emotions and emotional disorders. Above all, depression and anger harm the liver *qi* and block it so that it can not flow freely (ibid. 12) (see Fig. 6). Symptoms identified as a consequence of pathogenic liver change are, for example: dizziness (*xuanyun* 眩晕), headache (*touteng* 头疼), insomnia (*bu mei* 不寐) or numbness (*mamu* 麻木) and many more (ibid. 12).

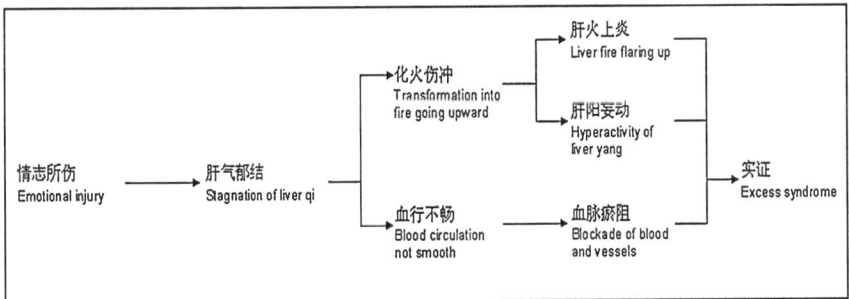

Fig. 6: *Pathogenesis of Liver Disease (segment) (Wang 2007a: 12).*

This textbook offers a broad overview of different case studies as well as more abstract descriptions of illness episodes, origins and treatments. As my own data reveals (see Chapter 6), depression is one of the most named illnesses of which the urban Chinese population thinks of as being caused by emotions. Therefore I use this book's chapter on depression (郁病) as an example of how it outlines the connections of emotions and illnesses. Depression is said to be caused mainly by an overreaction of emotions, which thereby acquire the possibility to be harmful to the organs ("郁病的主要病因为五志过极，七情内伤") (ibid. 262). Lasting irritations of emotions, especially of anger, unhappiness, sorrow, anxiety and thinking, injures the liver, causes its dysfunction and its failure to disperse *qi* properly, which then results in stagnation of liver *qi* and an insufficient flowing of blood. This leads to an acute excess syndrome, turning into a deficiency syndrome if protracted (ibid. 262) (Fig. 7). Depression is known for both sexes, but especially young and middle-aged women are, according to this textbook, in danger of suffering from it (ibid 263).[87]

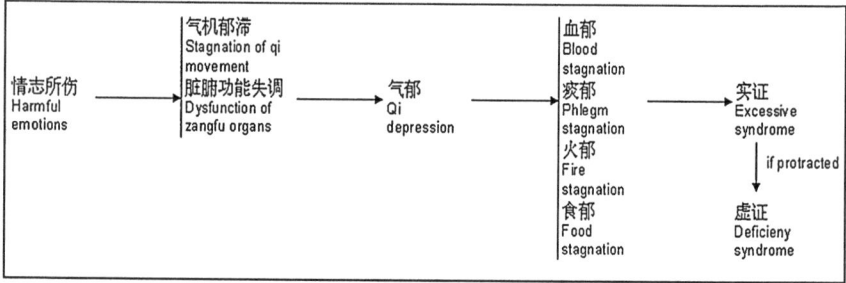

Fig. 7: Aetiology of Depression (segment) (Wang 2007a: 262).

In contrast to the other two books so far examined in this chapter, the *Zhongyi neikexue* points out that the therapeutic principle for curing emotion related diseases like depression are, besides the removal of blockades and excesses respec-

---

87   This corresponds with the findings by Phillips, Liu and Zhang (1999). In their article "Suicide and Social Change in China" they can reveal that China is one of the few countries in the world where women have a higher prevalence of committing suicide than men, at least until the end of the 1990s. I also refer to Hsieh & Spence (1980): they show that in pre-modern China a woman committing suicide, especially in order to implement loyalty to her family and her husband, was "presented as a model figure" (Hsieh & Spence 1980: 28). However, for my own data there is no significant difference in gender concerning the framing of depression as an emotion induced illness. Both sexes mentioned it equally (see Chapter 6).

tively deficiencies, to develop a peaceful and optimistic mood (ibid. 264). Patients should avoid strong emotional experiences and should exercise their body in order to strengthen their mind. Doctors are required to understand the patient's situation and to gain his or hers trust, so that the patient will be optimistic and his or her mood will change (ibid. 267).

Zhongyi linchuang jichu

The *Zhongyi linchuang jichu* (中医临床基础 "Clinical Basics of Traditional Chinese Medicine"), likewise published by Wang Xinyue (王新月, 2007b), frequently refers to the HDNJ while dealing with the pathogenic potential of emotions. It states that under normal conditions emotions are not dangerous, but emphasizes that if emotions occur too suddenly or are characterized as intense or prolonged, this leads to disturbed *qi* and blood, disorders of *yin* and *yang* and thereby provides possibilities for diseases to occur (ibid. 34). These illnesses are labelled "endogenous injuries due to the seven emotions" ("内伤七情") (ibid.).

The five emotions which are closely connected to the *zang*-organs may injure the corresponding organ directly. This is proved by a quotation of the HDNJ, referring to the same passage like the *Zhongyi jichu lilun*: "anger injures the liver, joy injures the heart, pensiveness injures the spleen, worry injures the lung, fear injures the kidney" – "怒伤肝，喜伤心，思伤脾，忧伤肺，恐伤肾"(ibid.).

Beside these direct relations, there are also more vague connections mentioned in this book. For example, excessive emotions may usually worsen a disease. On the other hand it is stated that open-minded, relaxed patients without strong emotionality may recover faster because of the harmonization of *qi* and blood and the five *zang*-organs (ibid.).

Contrary to the previously analysed book, the *Zhongyi linchuang jichu* focuses only on 'somatic' treatment of illnesses caused by emotions; renouncing 'psychological' approaches like developing a peaceful and optimistic mood. The chapter on '*Qi* up-rushing disease' for example recommends the therapeutic principle "clear heat and reverse the upward flow of *qi*, harmonizing blood and regulating liver" and adds a detailed prescription of eight herbal drugs, although it is said that this illness is often caused by emotional factors like fear, fright or anger (ibid. 242-243). To eliminate these emotional factors is not required according to this book. Hysteria (*zangzaobing* 脏躁病) is characterized as mainly related to emotional injury, emotional upset or excessive thinking. It will injure the liver and the heart and thereby leads to a deficiency syndrome. Therefore the therapeutic principle is to "treat deficiency by tonifying", but no 'counselling' or other; non soma-based treatment is recommended (ibid. 240).

The analysis of the selected textbooks reveals that emotions are consistently regarded as potentially pathogenic. All of the presented books show interdependence between specific organs and emotions respresenting a link between certain emotional states and specific illnesses. Nevertheless, when it comes to practice, most of the books refer to 'somatic' therapeutic interventions and aim at the 'somatic' manifestations.

5. Somatization: 'Eastern Culture-Bound Syndrome' or 'Western Culture-Bound Perspective'?

The analysis of the modern textbooks on Chinese medicine reveals that emotions are still perceived as an important etiological factor. These books state that emotions can cause a whole range of different diseases or worsen illnesses. However, when it comes to treatment, emotions in a [Western] psychological sense are more or less neglected. Only one of the selected textbooks (Wang 2007a) recommends developing a peaceful and optimistic mood and asks the doctor to gain the patient's trust in order to create a relaxed and calm atmosphere. The other treatment methods outlined in the analyzed textbooks all focus on 'somatic' treatment (i.e. on the prescription of herbal medicine which is supposed to eliminate the 'somatic' manifestations of the illnesses, the stagnations, blockades, deficiencies and excesses). They do not focus on changing the patient's inharmonious emotional condition by recommending 'psyche'-related treatment methods such as counselling, recommendations for changing the depressive or upsetting situation, or coping with sadness and sorrow. This coincides and corresponds with the patient's tendency to 'somatize' (i.e. primarily present 'somatic' symptoms while seeking 'psychological' help), which has been proven in the Chinese context in various observations such as the groundbreaking work of Arthur Kleinman (1979, 1982, 1986). He showed that between 80% and 90% of Chinese psychiatric outpatients from the 1950s to 1980 received the diagnosis of 'neurasthenia' (*shenjing shuairuo* 神经衰弱) instead of depression, which should have been the correct diagnosis according to DSM-III[88]. Neurasthenia is a disease concept that is coded as a nervous weakness mainly manifesting in somatic symptoms such as headache, loss of concentration, loss of appetite etc., and "confers far less stigma than [a diagnosis] of depression" (Lee & Kleinman 2007: 849). The term 'somatization' is used to

---

88 DSM = Diagnostic and Statistic Manual of Mental Disorders, published by the American Psychiatric Association. DSM-I was published in 1952, DSM-II in 1968. DSM-III was published in 1980, whereas DSM-IV was published in 1994. Currently, the Association is working on the newest version, DSM-V (see the homepage of the American Psychiatric Association www.psych.org and the homepage on DSM-V development www.dsm5.org).

describe a pattern of illness behaviour, especially a style of clinical presentation, in which somatic symptoms are presented to the exclusion or eclipse of emotional distress and social problems (Kirmayer & Young 1998: 420),

and that

although its prevalence and specific features vary considerably across cultures, the process of focussing on, amplifying, and clinically presenting somatic distress are universal and somatic symptoms are the most common clinical expression of emotional distress worldwide[89] (ibid.).

Lin et al. indicate it as the "chief idiom through which Chinese culture articulates [...] neurotic disorders" (Lin et al. 1980: 253, also see Kleinman 1979: 119-179). The term 'somatization' was criticized in cultural anthropology for implying the ethnocentric concept of a separation of soma and psyche. This leads to the accusation that non-Western societies, while referring to 'somatic' rather 'psychological' complaints, are mistaken, and that the usage of "psychological idioms [is] inherently more 'advanced' than somatic idioms" (Kirmayer & Young 1998: 426). Fabrega (1990b) calls it a "cultural and historical product of Western medicine" (653) based on a "quintessentially modern European biomedical epistemology" (654). It is functional as well as ontological as it presupposes physiological processes to be the root of illness and attributes illnesses "an existence and identity of their own" (Fabrega 1991: 182). So (2007) shows that 'somatizing' patients are "often dismissed as faking their symptoms" (168) and emphasizes that "non-biological events" (i.e. social and cultural context and the totality of the individual's life experience (172)), must be considered as influencing both the patient's and the doctor's explanatory model of illness.

Nevertheless, the research literature on Chinese medicine, especially concerning 'psychological' issues, is overflowing with case studies showing the strategy of 'somatization' (in additional to the already mentioned works of Kleinman from the 1980s more recent publications are for example Ots 1999: 33-36, Park &

---

89 Beside China, 'somatization' has been observed in diverse countries and societies, for example in India (Sethi 1986, Rao 2007), in the United Arab Emirates (Hamdi et al. 1997), in Colombia (Escobar 1983) and also among migrants from turkey living in Germany (Üresim 2008). In this light one could actually say with Kleinman that "it is not somatization but psychologization in the Western middle and upper class that is unusual and requires explanation" (Kleinman 1986: 56).

Hinton 2002: 229-231, Zhang 2007b: 79-80 etc.). Generally, 'somatization' is thought of as allowing individuals to perform the sick role – which in certain societies is socially more accepted – instead of the stigmatized deviant role of the mentally ill (Ryder et al. 2008: 302, c.f. Goldberg & Bridges 1988: 142-143). This is particularly true for the Chinese. Chinese patients during consultation commonly present 'somatic' complains and the doctors routinely refer to 'somatic' processes. For Ots (1990) and other scholars (Kleinman 1979, Tseng & Wu 1985, and Bond 1993), there exists "a long standing tradition of repression of emotions [...] mainly based on Neo-Confucian ideals", whereas "emotional excess is highly stigmatized" (Ots 1990: 25).[90] Therefore, both patients and doctors, avoid talking straightforward about emotional problems but address the treatment directly to the internal, 'somatic' conditions (c.f. Wu 1982: 292).[91]

During the Cultural Revolution in China (1966-1976), this stigmatization was even intensified as emotional problems were seen as problems of wrong political attitude for a 'true' and 'confident' socialist could *per definitionem* not be distressed or depressed (Chang et al. 2005: 105).[92] Tung (1994) emphasizes that the Chinese self-conception is "primarily social and interpersonal" and is "concerned with constant judgement of one's being good or bad, right or wrong" (488). When emotional equilibrium is a requested condition, emotional disorder is a violation of this demand and thus is offending to the social context of the individual, as "[being] fundamentally a part of a larger whole" (490). Also, more recent studies into emotional disorders (for example Lu et al. 2008, Zane & Yev 2002) stress the importance of support by the social group and the family and

---

90   East Asian societies are said to be denying and suppression emotions, as the display of emotions in social interaction can be judged as weakness and threat to social harmony (Kawanishi 1992: 7). From my own experience, I acknowledge this, but on the other hand I indicate that from this characterization it is only a hairbreadth to common cliché on East Asian societies. Thus, among other stereotypes, Shen et al. (2011) identified passiveness, obedience and lack of emotional expression as common clichés (283, 291). For further reading on the connection between stereotyping, discrimination and mental health issues among East Asian populations I refer to Lin & Cheung (1999) and to Spencer et al. (2010).

91   Messner (2006) shows that even in the classical book Huandi Neijing „the differentiation between physical appearance (xing 形) and the mood/feeling/emotions (zhi 志) appearance seems of little or no importance if we concentrate on the advice given for treatment. Of all the five methods mentioned there is not even one that does not focus on the concrete body (Messner 2006: 56).

92   I further refer to Pearson (1995) for a concise overview about the history of mental health care in China, not only during the Cultural Revolution, but from the end of the empire until the implementation of the opening policy during the early 1990s.

the integration of the individual into the social context, which the Chinese individual would endanger through confessing emotional instability.[93]

Thus, is 'somatization' a common feature of Chinese medicine and Chinese society? Or more generally, is 'somatization' an Eastern culture-bound syndrome, as especially the older research literature states, or a Western culture-bound perspective, because Western biomedicine coined the term[94] and Western psychology rendered a diagnostic framework for it? It is not a specifically non-Western syndrome at all; for example, it is estimated that 10 percent of all medical treatment in the United States is delivered to patients presenting somatic symptoms without any evidence of organic diseases, costing $20 billion annually (Smith 2009: 1). And Zhou et al. (2011) prove in a cross-cultural analysis that Chinese do not in every situation tend to 'somatize'. Instead Euro-Canadians during specific illness episodes have a higher tendency to 'somatize'; for example, while suffering from anxiety disorders. As the empirically evidence proves, 'somatization' is much more common around the world than "psychologization" (the counter-term, which White coined in 1982).

There is some evidence that the tendency to 'somatize' is not, in the first place, a culture-bound or 'cultural', but rather a social and economic phenomenon. Kleinman and Kleinman show that the presentation of 'somatic' symptoms was the normal way of dealing with 'psychological' diseases in Western societies for a long time, until in the "Victorian middle class" influenced by a "cultural transformation shaped by modernism [...] a deeper interiorization of the self has been constituted" (Kleinman & Kleinman 2007: 470). This led to the diagnosis of 'somatization' when patients complained about 'somatic' symptoms while the 'true' cause of the disorder was thought of as being part of the 'psyche' (ibid.). Consequently, from their point of view, Western middle class individuals shape 'affects' as deep psychological experience and tend to rationalize it into classified emotions like depression, anger or anxiety, which leads to the conclusion that both; 'somatization' as well as 'psychologization' are "cultural construc-

---

93 Social harmony is valued in other East Asian societies, too. In Japanese, there exist the terms gaman (我慢) and gamanzuyoi (我慢強い) which covers a broad range of meanings starting with "patience" and ending with "endurance in the face of hardship". It is one of the main virtues that were taught to Japanese children in order to cultivate and respect social harmony (Kawanishi 1992: 7).

94 Smith (2009: 2) shows that the Austrian psychoanalyst Wilhelm Stekel (1868-1940) invented the term in the 1920s, when he was quarrelling with Sigmund Freud (1856-1939) about the correct direction of psychoanalysis.

tions of psychobiological processes" (ibid. 471). Kawanishi (1992: 5) reveals that "lower class, less educated populations" are believed to 'somatize' more, and Woolfolk & Allan (2007: 33) present data that 'somatizers' in an American setting are more likely to be unemployed and less productive than patients presenting 'psychological' symptoms.[95] This hint to the connection between modernism, the emerging middle class and 'psychologization' is an interesting track which I would like to follow in the interpretation of my own data (see Chapter 7). It opens a door for speculation regarding the stigma of somatic or psychological complains. When a society begins to regard stress due to an exhausting, responsible job as an achievement, an overflowing appointment calendar as a means of social integration and importance and the 'bureau-in-the-pocket' as providing one with full-time approachableness, but the same society regards 'somatic' problems as a lack of proper caring for the body by mixing an unhealthy lifestyle with laziness and weakness, the stigma of emotion-induced illnesses is prone to decrease whereas bodily illnesses are, at least partially, maybe coded as self-induced.

Nevertheless and admitting all the problems that surround the term 'somatization', it has a certain descriptive quality, pointing to the fact that a specific category of symptoms is presented (i.e. 'somatic' ones) and another category of symptoms is neglected. Of course, this can only be recognized with the biomedical bias that features the separation of body and mind and hosts the concept of 'somatization'. Therefore I use this term descriptively and tagged with apostrophes to reveal the problematic dimensions of this term and of course acknowledging that this is an etic point of view.[96]

The problems with this term can be contained at least to a certain degree: I demonstrate that for Chinese professionals of Chinese medicine the two categories of 'somatic' and 'psychological' symptoms exist, too. Cosequently, these medical experts are used to both kinds of patient's complains, 'somatic' as well as 'psychological'. All of my expert interviewees used this differentiation between 'body' (*shenti* 身体) and 'psyche' (*xinli* 心理) in order to denominate different categories of symptoms. From their point of view, both manifestations are

---

95 The rather old study by Merskey and Spear (1967) reveals as well that in a Western clinical setting people from a lower socio-economic background and larger families are especially somatically focused and presenting painful, 'somatic' symptoms (c.f. Chaturvedi et al. 2006: 76-77).

96 Furthermore I do not impose any evolutionistic or judgemental implications in my usage of this term. It is just used to describe that some patients with emotion-related illnesses present symptoms which are biomedically spoken related to the somatic sphere.

correct, for they hold that emotional distress and emotion-induced illnesses can manifest in both 'somatic' and 'psychological' ways.

6. Empirical Results

In the preceding chapters, I demonstrated that Chinese philosophical thought has constructed a close interdependence between human emotions and illnesses by embedding it in a broader concept of macrocosmic and microcosmic harmony. When human emotions are in excess, this harmony is endangered and illnesses may arise. Based on this philosophical concept, Chinese classical medical texts draw close connections between emotions and the human body, postulating direct interconnectedness of emotional instability and human organs. Recent medical texts on Chinese medicine corroborate these ideas and specify a set of emotions with high pathological potential. In this chapter, I shall present empirical data revealing the attitudes and the knowledge of Chinese urban dwellers concerning Chinese medicine in general and concerning the relationship between emotions and health in detail; the data will be followed by interpretation and discussion, followed up by analysis in chapter seven.

I collected empirical data with two different methodological approaches. First I conducted a questionnaire survey and gathered merely quantitative data, although many conversations with the informants developed into informal interviews providing me with rich additional material. The survey questionnaire (see appendix 1) contains 27 questions and 16 statements which the participants were asked either to reject or to approve.

Moreover, beside this quantitative approach I also conducted semi-structured interviews with medical experts to acquire qualitative data. I conducted 20 comprehensive interviews with experts in Chinese medicine, among them 12 doctors, three members of hospital staff, four students of Chinese medicine and one clinic manager. The students were all enrolled at the Beijing University of Chinese medicine (北京中医药大学), the hospital staff was working in three different hospitals in the city centre of Beijing. These three hospitals had different characteristics. The first one was a small size outpatient clinic mainly treating disorders that would be denoted as stress-related or psychosomatic in biomedical context, using mainly acupuncture and moxibustion and focusing on a middle class clientele. The second clinic was a mid-sized clinic and open to a broader public, but also commonly frequented by so called 'white collar workers' of the surrounding offices. Different "famous doctors"[97] had their weekly consultation hours there and it was supplied with a build-in pharmacy selling Chinese medicines. The third clinic was a big hospital located south of the city

---

97 Quotation of the clinic manager.

centre, one of the main treatment and research institutions of Chinese medicine in whole China.[98]

In this chapter, I first present the results of the questionnaire survey, then subsequently discuss these results and afterwards I delineate the results of the informal interviews with medical experts.

The Questionnaire Survey

As already pointed out in more detail in chapter two, the survey was carried out in residential neighbourhoods in the city centre of Beijing, in 'small neighbourhoods' or *xiaoqu* (小区), where I asked people living in this area if they were willing to fill in the questionnaire. I investigated in the *Haidian* District (海淀区) around the streets *Haidian nanlu* (海淀南路) and *Suzhoujie* (苏州街) as well as in the *Zhongguancun* shopping centre(中关村), in the *Fengtai* District (丰台区) in the vicinity of the *Liujiayao* subway station (刘家窑站), which was the local people's emic label for this particular quarter, in *Dongcheng* District (东城区) in the *Hutongs* (胡同) surrounding the drum tower and bell tower, and in *Chaoyang* District (朝阳区) especially in the area close to the *Guomao* bridge (国贸桥) (see Fig. 8).

---

98 For a closer description of the clinics see chapter 6 and appendix 3.

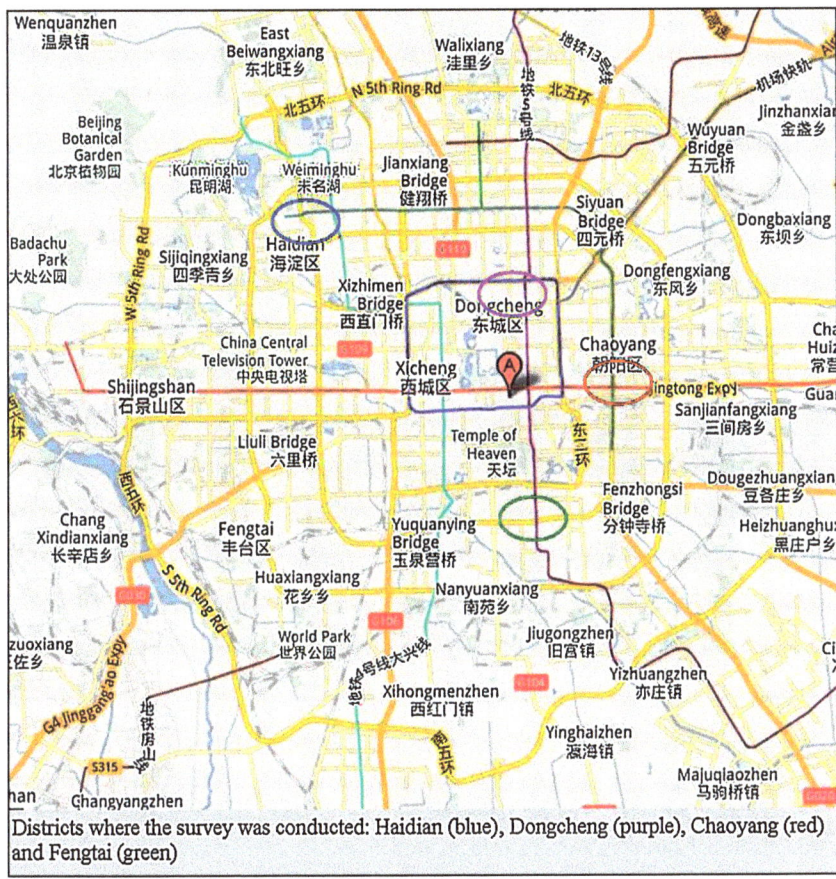

Districts where the survey was conducted: Haidian (blue), Dongcheng (purple), Chaoyang (red) and Fengtai (green)

Fig. 8: *Investigation areas (Google maps, own modifications). Hadian district and Zhongguancun shopping mall (blue circle), Dongcheng district and hutongs (purple circle), Chaoyang district (red circle) and Fengtai disctrict with the quarter Liujiayao (green circle).*

In total 253, people participated in the survey: 134 were women and 119 were men. For further analysis, I divided the sample in different age cohorts and according to level of education and economical background (see appendix 2). For my sample I tried to maintain a more or less balanced gender-ratio throughout the different age groups (see Fig. 9). In the *Haidian* District around the streets *Suzhoujie* and *Haidian nanlu*, I asked 35 people to participate and at the *Zhongguancun* shopping centre, which is also located in the *Haidian* District, 34 people participated in the survey. In the *Dongcheng* District I questioned 70 inhabitants while in *Chaoyang* 50 respondents were engaged and in *Fengtai*, 47 people answered my questions (see Fig. 10).

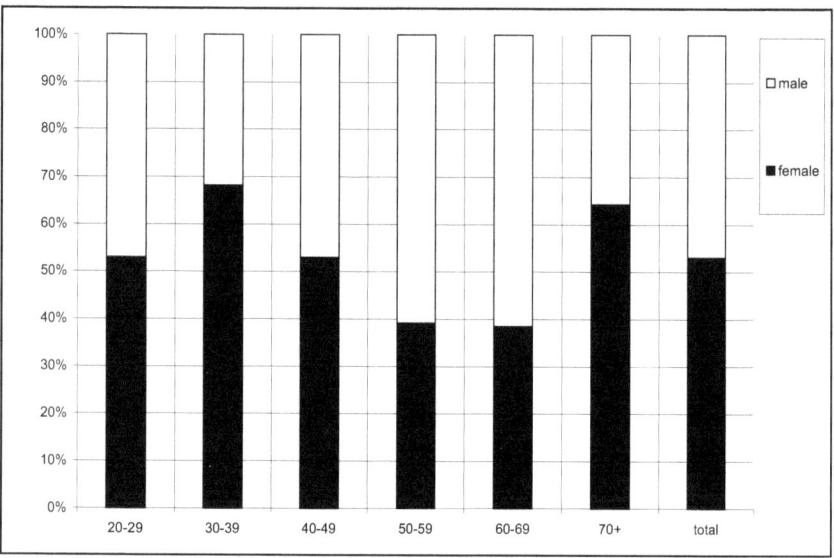

Fig. 9: *Distribution of gender in age groups among survey participants (Böke: Fieldwork 2010/2011).*

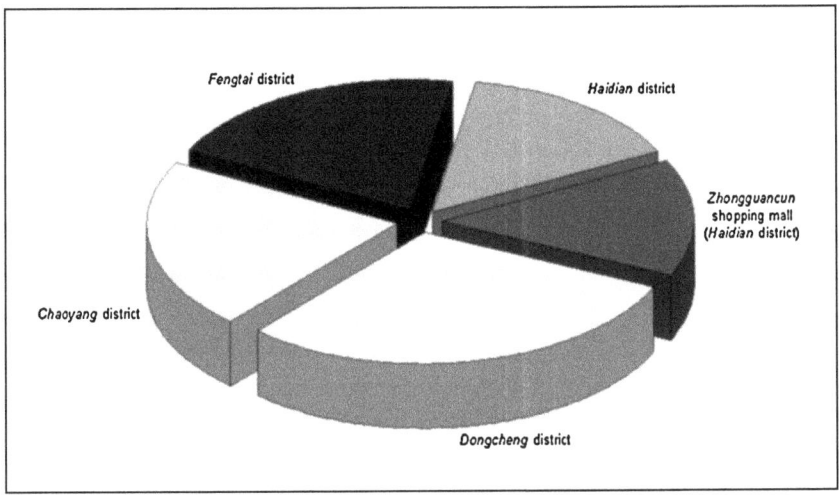

Fig. 10: *Distribution of survey participants according to city districts (Böke: Fieldwork 2010/2011).*

Construction of the Questionnaire

The questions were constructed with three different answering categories: the first category consists of dichotomous variables ('yes-or-no-questions'). The second is characterized by polytomous variables, where the informants had to choose between different answers by ticking the appropriate box. The third kind of answer category is open-ended which leave space for people's own ideas and attitudes beyond the firmly imposed categories. The questions can be further clustered into different categories regarding their content. First, there are questions about participant's general evaluations in the context of health and illness (for example: 'Do emotions cause illnesses?'). Secondly, participants were asked about their knowledge of certain concepts in Chinese medicine ('Do you know the term Six Evils?'), accompanied with the question about the meaning of this term ('What is the meaning of Six Evils?'). The last section consists of self-reporting questions ('Where did you get your knowledge about Chinese medicine?').

The statements which had to be approved or rejected are clustered into five blocks. First, there are statements concerning medical relationships ('Emotions can influence health'). Additionally a second block deals with evaluations

('Chinese medicine works better than Western medicine'). A third category asks more concrete about the pathogenic potential of emotions ('Emotions can affect organs'), whereas a fourth section deals with the evaluation of indigenous concepts ('The Six Evils are an important etiological category'). The last block names alternatives for action ('If someone suffers from emotional instability, he/she should visit a psychotherapist').

The Percept Pathological Potential of Emotions

Regarding the first section of the questionnaire concerning general evaluations in the context of health and illness, there is a broad consensus that emotions can cause illness; 97% of the participants affirm this question (see Fig. 11) and consequently, variations according to age group, gender, education or economic status can not be detected.

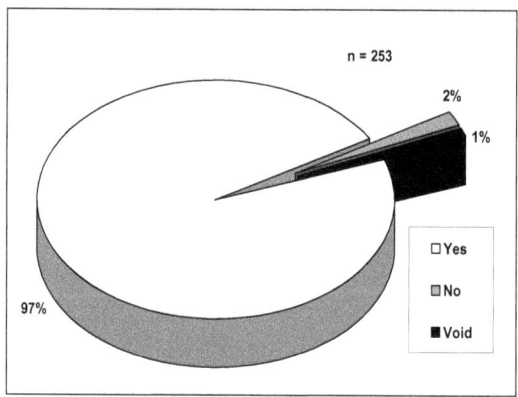

Fig. 11: *Can emotions induce illnesses? (Böke: Fieldwork 2010/2011).*

Hence emotions are not only perceived as etiological factors in Chinese philosophy and classical medical texts as well as in recently published Chinese textbooks; the urban population also shares this view with astonishing conformance.

Looking at the specific illnesses which are thought of as being caused by emotions, I collected in total 458 statements. Among them, one can identify a tendency to emphasize heart illnesses (*xinzangbing* 心脏病), which are most frequently named as being caused by emotions. The second most named illness in this context is depression (*yiyuzheng* 抑郁症), followed up by 'insanity' (*jingshenbing* 精神病) and high blood pressure (*gaoxueya* 高血压). Additionally, stomach problems (*weibing* 胃病), *neifenmi* (内分泌)[99] and liver disease (*ganbing* 肝病) were mentioned frequently (see Fig. 12).

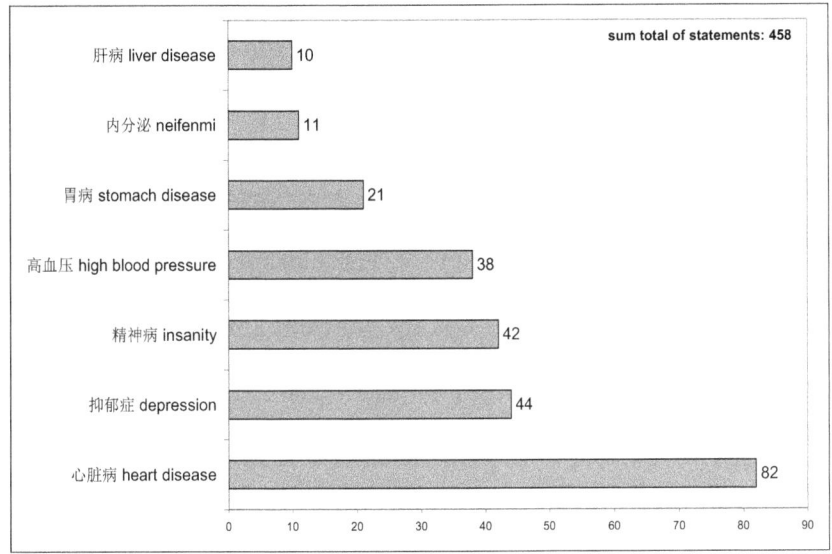

***Fig. 12**: Most frequently mentioned illness terms (at least named ten times) (Böke: Fieldwork 2010/2011).*

Although at first glance the distribution of all the named illnesses seems to be quite homogenous and forms mainly the two categories of heart related illnesses (heart disease and high blood pressure) and psychological issues (depression and 'insanity'), indeed there are more than 50 illness terms which were only mentioned once. Hence, aside from these two rather homogenous sectors of heart diseases and psychological issues, there is a vast heterogeneity in the distribution of illnesses perceived as caused by emotions in Chinese urban population. This extensive list covers more severe illnesses from every branch of medicine;

---

[99] Which literally means 'endocrine gland'. It refers to an acupuncture point which is commonly used in treating anxiety disorders (Liu et al. 2012, Pilkington et al. 2007, Wang et al. 2001).

for example autism, cancer or pneumonia, but also comparatively minor health problems such as indigestion, insomnia or headache (not listed in Fig. 12).

Under a gendered lens, one finds the general tendency of women to answer in more detailed and to give more of a variety of illness terms than men. On average, each male participant only named 1.6 illness terms, whereas each female participant named 2.0 terms. Eleven men, but only three women did not specify any illness. This coincides with my impression during the fieldwork that women were more interested in this topic. Furthermore, they reported more openly, even about personal or interfamilial health issues.

However, significantly different answering patterns can be observed if one evaluates the statements referring to illnesses caused by emotions according to age groups. Then one finds decidedly generation-specific answers. Whereas older generations mainly named heart disease or high blood pressure and completely neglected 'psychological' issues such as depression, younger people mainly identified these 'psychological' issues and presented a much broader range of illness terms in this particular field than their older cohorts.[100] Accordingly, among the participants which were older than 70, no one mentioned depression (*yiyuzheng* 抑郁症) or other related terms as being caused by emotions. From the 19 answers collected in this age group, heart disease and blood pressure alone take up ten. In addition, insanity was listed three times with six other illness terms only listed once. For the age group of 60 to 69 years, one can identify a similar pattern. Out of a total of 16 answers, heart disease with three answers is the only term listed more than once. For the youngest age group engaged in the survey, people aged between 20 and 29, depression is the most commonly mentioned illness, expressed in the five terms *yiyuzheng* (抑郁症), *youyuzheng* (忧郁症), *yumen* (郁闷), *youmen* (忧闷) and the more colloquial term *kongxiangzheng* (恐想症). These terms total an amount of 29 answers, whereas heart disease with 25 answers and insanity with 16 answers occupy second and third position. Significantly, not only is depression the most commonly named illness associated with emotions amongst the youngest survey participants, but the semantic field of terms denoting depression-related illnesses is represented as much more differentiated here than in any other age group.

---

100 For the sample and cohort sizes see appendix 2.

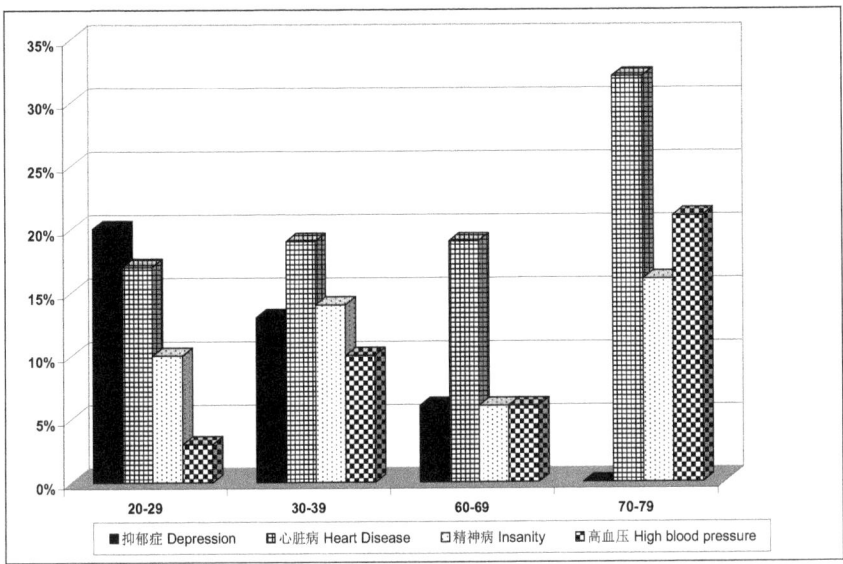

Fig. 13a*: Illnesses caused by emotions: age-specific answering patterns (most commonly named illnesses in percentage) (Böke: Fieldwork 2010/2011).*

According to these findings it can be estimated that among younger urban Chinese, depression, with its different Chinese terms, is more significant than among older inhabitants. With increasing age, the mentioning of depression decreases, ending in the total absence in the answers of the oldest participants (see Fig. 13a). Simultaneously with the quantitative decrease in numbers, a qualitative decrease in the complexity of the semantic field can be observed. Whereas the youngest age group differentiated five different terms meaning depression, the following two age groups (30 to 39 years and 40 to 49 years) only named two terms, *yiyuzheng* (抑郁症) and *youyuzheng* (忧郁症). The 50 to 59 year old participants only named the one term *yiyuzheng* (抑郁症), whereas the 60 to 69 year old only listed the term *youyuzheng* (忧郁症).

Considering the different sample sizes, the age cohorts 60-69 only covers 13 individuals, the cohort 70+ covers only 14; they were combined to create an age group 60 and older with 27 individuals to enhance comparability. However, this construction does not seriously change the results (Fig 13b) but supports the findings of age-specific answering patterns: the stronger emphasis of heart-related issues like heart disease and high blood pressure among the older urban population, and the stronger emphasis of 'psychological issues', especially with regard to depression, among the younger population.

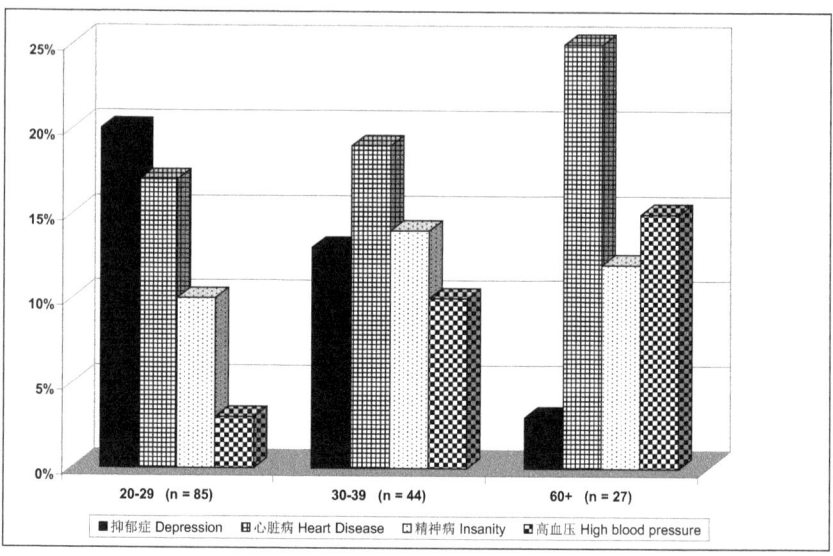

Fig. 13b: Illnesses caused by emotions: age-specific answering patterns (most commonly named illnesses in percentage) (Böke: Fieldwork 2010/2011).

At this point I continue to present the survey results, but will return to discuss this answering behaviour in more detailed later on in this chapter.

The Relationship Between Organs and Emotions

Similar to the conformity about the etiological potential of emotions, one finds a broad consensus about the influence of emotions on the *zangfu*-organ system[101]. To the question of whether emotions can directly influence the *zangfu*, 96% agreed that emotions could have an influence, with only 3% rejecting this. As only 1% made no statement or stated uncertainty, one can assume that there is a far-reaching consensus among the Chinese urban population about the direct

---

101   For more information on the zangfu see Chapter 1.

connection between emotions and organs, a connection which is – as already shown – also outlined in the different texts and books on Chinese medicine. Again one finds congruence between expert knowledge written in specialists' books and the attitudes of common urban residents. Looking closer, I asked about the relationships between specific *zangfu*-organs and specific emotions. First, the organs 'liver' (*gan* 肝) and heart (*xin* 心) were identified in particular as being susceptible to influence by emotions (Fig 14).

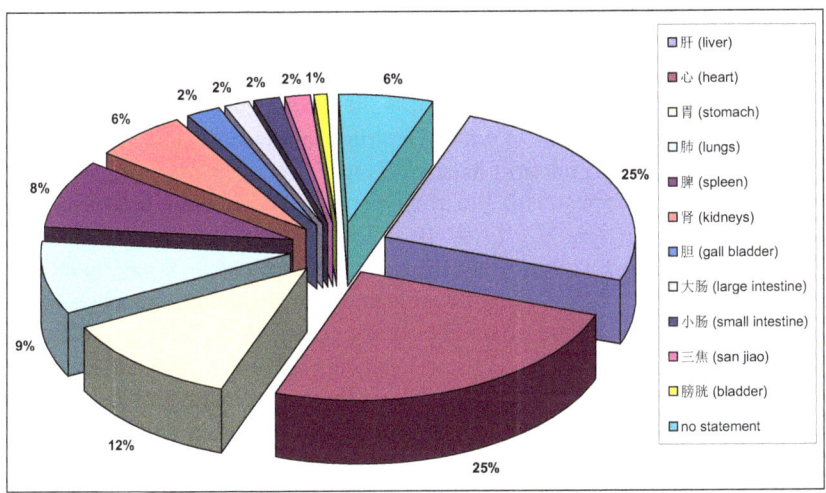

Fig. 14: Organs perceived as being potentially influenced by emotions (Böke: Fieldwork 2010/2011).

Exactly half of the connections between emotions and organs drawn by my informants referred to these two organs. The 'stomach' (*wei* 胃) was named in 12% of the answers, whereas the rest of the *zangfu*-organs only acquired monadic results. Only 6% of the answers were unspecific. As multiple answers were possible, this equals approximately 10% of all participants. Consequently, 90% of the interviewees dared to give specific answers. According to the theory of Chinese medicine and as shown in chapters three and four, every organ is connected to a specific emotion and – at least theoretically – is prone to be influenced by it. But like in some texts of Chinese medical theory (see chapter 4), where the heart and the liver are mentioned most frequently and other organs like bladder or the intestines are almost neglected, the lay perspective also concentrates on heart and liver and estimates these organs to be especially vulnerable to emotional influence.

Focusing on the second part of the question, one finds a great number of emotions as potentially pathologic. In total, given that multiple answers were possible, 118 different emotion terms were mentioned by the survey participants, many of these terms were named only once. The most common terms were *shengqi* (生气) and *nu* (怒), both meaning 'anger', which cover about 35% of all statements. Every other term only reached monadic values.

These two findings, first the significance of heart and liver as organs perceived to be easily affected by emotions, and second, the crucial role of 'anger' represented in the two terms *shengqi* (生气) and *nu* (怒) as carrying special pathologic potential, meet in the description of the connection between organs and emotions. The interviewees most often mentioned connection between a specific organ and a specific emotion was the connection between 'liver' (*gan* 肝) and 'anger' (*shengqi* 生气) with 31 entries, followed by the connection between liver and the second term meaning 'anger' (*nu* 怒), with 30 entries. Still quite significant is the accumulation of the perceived connection between 'heart' (*xin* 心) and 'anger' (*nu* 怒), listed 19 times, and between heart and 'anger' (*shengqi* 生气), listed 11 times. Furthermore, multiple other connections were mentioned, but with pronounced heterogeneity and without statistical significance. In summary, Chinese urban population perceives the *zangfu*-organs 'liver' (*gan* 肝) and 'heart' (*xin* 心) as seriously susceptible to influence by emotions belonging to the anger-complex. While there is a broad consensus regarding this connection, the connections between further organs and emotions are perceived as much more heterogeneous. The same is true for emotions potentially influencing the organs: aside from the consensus concerning the emotions 'anger' (*shengqi* 生气and *nu* 怒) and the organs 'liver' (*gan*肝) and heart (*xin*心), there is extreme heterogeneity. At least partially, these results mirror the expert's estimation as presented both in the classical and modern writings of Chinese medicine. Through the ages, anger has been indicated as specifically harmful, and the liver and the heart are described as organs which are especially prone to be influenced by emotions.

The Knowledge of Chinese Medical Concepts

The second set of questions can be summarized as relating to theoretical knowledge. I asked about the familiarity with the Chinese medical concepts of the 'Five Phases', the 'Six Evils' and the 'Seven Emotion'[102] and about the

---

102 For a concise overview about these concepts see Chapter 1.

recognition of the book HDNJ[103]. This book, which is still quoted in contemporary textbooks and routinely referred to by Chinese doctors in medical examinations, is known in the urban population, although with some limitations (see Fig. 15). Even if almost two-thirds of the participants have at least heard of it, less than 20% were confident enough to answer straightforward that they know it. The majority chose to answer more vaguely and said that they have heard of the book on some occasion. Commonly, in the dialogue around this question, people who answered that they know the HDNJ either told me that they gathered their knowledge concerning this book from television shows with medical content or that they know it from explanations by the doctor.

When asked whether this book is relevant, almost half of the participants stated that it is relevant and only 10% said that they do not think it is relevant. A rather high amount of respondents made no statement, which shows that many of the interviewed persons who stated that they had heard of this book must not have been familiar with its contents and its focus; they were not able to estimate its relevance. The common reasons why it was rated relevant were that it is an important book of Chinese medicine used by doctors and that it is a collection of important ancient knowledge. The other position was mainly characterized as calling the book outdated and obsolete. Additionally, some interviewees responded that it is a specialist book for practitioners of Chinese medicine and therefore irrelevant for common people.

---

103 For an analysis of this book see Chapter 3

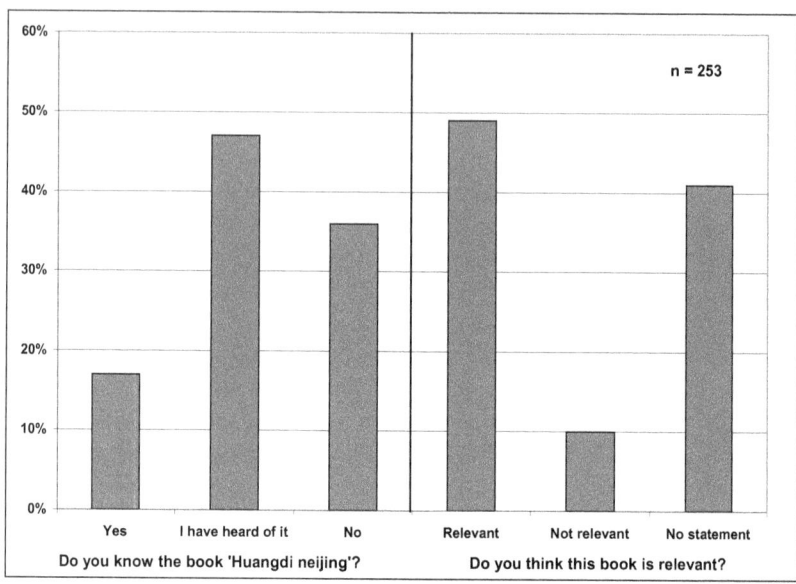

Fig. 15: Knowledge and evaluation of the book 'Huangdi neijing' (Böke: Fieldwork 2010/2011).

Summarizing one can say that there is knowledge of the HDNJ, although hazy in many cases. I could not observe any relevant differences in the answers along demographic lines. Evidently, the better educated the respondents, the higher was the likelihood that they knew or had heard of this book. The perceived relevance, though, was not significantly influenced by educational background.

The other observations concerning knowledge of medical concepts reveal an interesting distribution. They show that the knowledge of standard concepts in Chinese medicine is not shared equally among Chinese urban population. As already analysed, the two main etiological categories of Chinese medicine are the 'Six Evils' (*liu xie* 六邪) and the 'Seven Emotions' (*qi qing* 七情). According to Chinese medical theory, all illness causes can be classified in one of these two categories (with the exception of separate descrete phenomena such as accidental injury, excessive labour, etc.). The model which connects these illness categories to organs and other bodily tissues is the system of the 'Five Phases' (*wuxing xueshuo* 五行学说)[104]. It is the standard model of bodily processes in Chinese medical theory. So by asking about the 'Five Phases', the 'Six Evils' and the 'Seven Emotions', I asked about concepts that are doubtlessly fundamental to Chinese medicine. However, the answers were quite diverse (see Fig. 16).

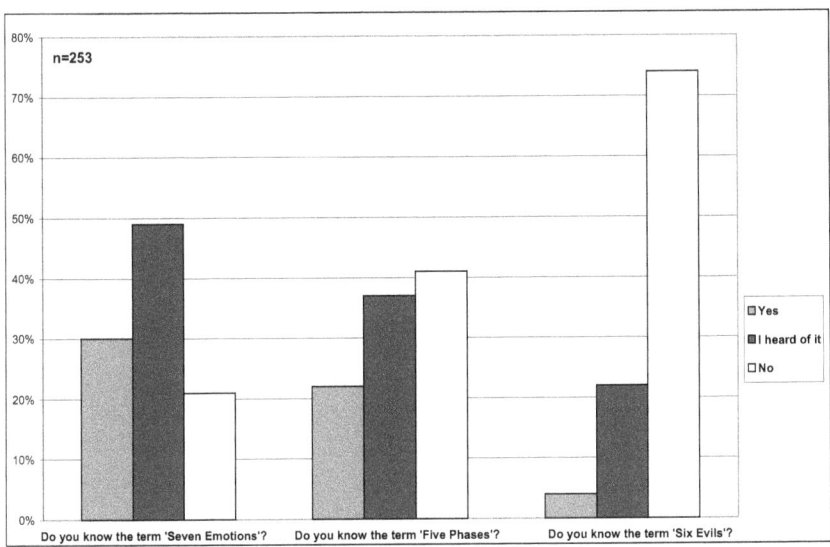

Fig. 16: *Self-reported knowledge of certain Chinese medical concepts (Böke: Fieldwork 2010/2011).*

The concept of the 'Seven Emotions' was the best-know of the three concepts, with almost 80% indicating that they either knew this term or had heard of it. The concept of the 'Five Phases' was lesser known among the investigated population; less than 60% knew this term or had heard of it. The concept of 'Six Evils' was mostly unknown among the interviewees with almost 80% reporting that they had never heard this term before. Differentiation according to educational background reveals that graduates from universities or colleges had a significant higher tendency to answer that they know the terms than people with intermediate school degree, whereas these people in turn were more likely to know these terms than people with primary school education (Fig. 17).

---

104 For an explanation of the 'Five Phases', the 'Six Evils' and the 'Seven Emotions' see Chapter 1.

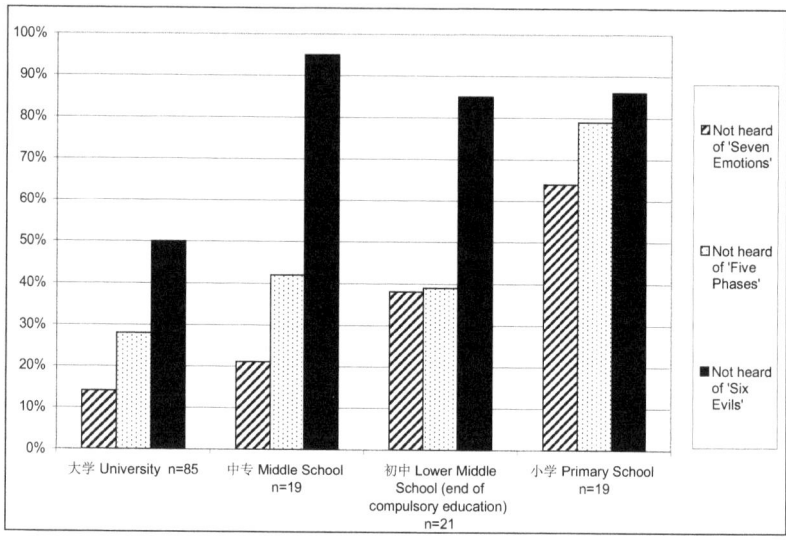

Fig. 17: Self-reported lack of knowledge of Chinese medical concepts according to education (Böke: Fieldwork 2010/2011).

Looking closer at the ideas which the urban population associate with these terms, I analyse the reported content or meaning of these different terms by starting with the best-known concept, the 'Seven Emotions', followed by the 'Five Phases' and ending with the 'Six Evils'.

Even if the term 'Seven Emotions' was the best known among interviewees, 38% (97 participants) could not specify this term and did not answer the question regarding the meaning of it. Interviewees answered to this question in almost all cases by listing different emotions. The most common answer however was the enumeration of the four emotions happiness, anger, grief and joy (*xi* 喜, *nu* 怒, *ai* 哀, *le* 乐). This answer was given 50 times, and many participants almost reflexively listed these emotion terms. It is probable that at least some of the interviewees used the expression of *xi, nu, ai, le* (喜, 怒, 哀, 乐) as a *pars pro toto* for emotionality as opposed to a list of specific emotions the informants associate with the medical concept of the 'Seven Emotions. The phrase (*qiqing liuyu* 七情六欲) was mentioned 31 times; it also means 'emotions' and is literally comprised of the medical paradigm of 'Seven Emotions' (*qi qing* 七情) and the notion of 'Six Desires' (*liu yu* 六欲) rooted in (Chinese) Buddhism. In contrast, most interviewees reported individual lists of emotion terms composing this lists out of a broad variety of terms.

An overview of the mentioned emotion terms reveals that some emotions are usually thought more of being part of the concept of 'Seven Emotions' than others (Fig. 18).

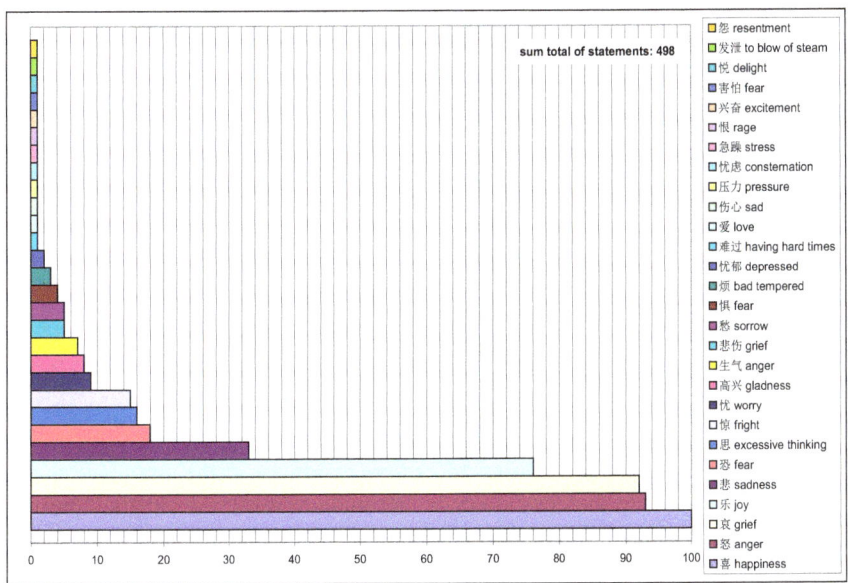

Fig. 18: *Numbers of emotions named as belonging to the 'Seven Emotions' (Böke: Fieldwork 2010/2011).*

Altogether, 29 different emotion terms were named, out of which 12 emotions were mentioned only once. The most commonly named emotions, which have already been mentioned above, were happiness, anger, grief and joy (*xi* 喜 , *nu* 怒 , *ai* 哀 , *le* 乐) with 100, 93, 92 and 76 entries respectively[105]. Emotions such as 'sadness' (*bei* 悲 , 33 entries), 'fear' (*kong* 恐 , 18 entries), 'excessive thinking' (*si* 思 , 16 entries), 'fright' (*jing* 惊 , 15 entries) and 'worry' (*you*忧 , eight

---

105 However, as explained above, one has to keep in mind that these numbers can be influenced by the fact that some informants supposedly used the phrase 喜, 怒, 哀, 乐 (xi nu ai le) not mainly as a list of emotion terms but as a more general expression simply meaning emotion.

entries) were also mentioned. The Seven Emotions, according to Chinese medical theory (*xi* 喜 , *nu* 怒 , *you* 忧 , *si* 思 , *bei* 悲 , *kong* 恐 and *jing* 惊) are all represented among the most commonly named terms, although the number of times they appear is significantly different. Compared to the question regarding the pathologic quality of emotions presented above, two findings are striking: first, a much lower diversity of emotion terms can be detected; and second, there is a different composition of emotion terms here. Thus, the Beijing urban population considers many more emotions to be pathologic than just those belonging to the category of 'Seven Emotions'. I discuss these findings more detailed in subchapter 6.1.4.2.

Regarding the meaning of the term 'Five Phases', more than half of the interviewees did not make any statement. Out of 254 questionnaires, 159 contained unspecific answers as wells as fuzzy and illegible writing. Nevertheless, 81 participants listed the five elements 'gold' (*jin* 金), 'wood' (*mu* 木), 'water' (*shui* 水), 'fire' (*huo* 火) and 'earth' (*tu* 土). According to Chinese medical theory, these elements name and identify the different 'phases'. A few people identified a connection to the concepts of *yin* and *yang*, to *Taiji* (太极)[106] or to astrology.

For the concept of the 'Six Evils' one has to state that it is almost unknown among the investigated population. More than two thirds of the interviewees did not give a response to the question of the meaning of this term. Only six participants listed the climatic influences 'wind' (*feng* 风), 'cold' (*han* 寒), 'summerheat' (*shu* 暑), 'dampness' (*shi* 湿), 'dryness' (*zao* 燥) and 'fire' (*huo* 火), which, according to Chinese medical theory, are the specific exogenous pathogenic factors labelled with the term 'Six Evils'. Some participants only listed one or two of these climatic influences whereas others gave miscellaneous answers like 'six kinds of illnesses in Chinese medicine' (*zhongyili de liu zhong bing* 中医里的六种病) or 'six kinds of unhealthy manners' (*liu zhong bu hao de xingwei* 六种不好的行为); these vague responses could not be further explained by the informants.

---

106 Taiji is a philosophical principle in Chinese philosophy and can be translated as 'Supreme Ultimate'. Zhang & Ryden (2002) explain this term by reference to the philosophical text 'Book of Change' (yijing 易经 / 易經): "Any philosophy that asserts two elements such as the yin-yang of Chinese philosophy will also look for a term to reconcile the two, to ensure that both belong to the same sphere of discourse. The term 'supreme ultimate' performs this role in the philosophy of the Book of Changes. In the Song dynasty it became a metaphysical term on a par with the Way" (179).

Concluding, one can say that there is a certain familiarity with basic concepts of Chinese medicine among Beijing urban population. However, this familiarity is not distributed equally; the concept of 'Seven Emotions', one of the two etiological categories of Chinese medicine, is best known. Approximately 80% stated that they either know this term or had heard of it. More than 60% could specify its meaning by listing specific emotions subsumed in this concept. Among the most commonly listed emotions, the 'correct' terms according to Chinese medical theory were represented. Contrary, the second etiological category in Chinese medicine, the 'Six Evils', is mostly unknown. Less than 30% of the survey participants are acquainted with this term and consequently, approximately 70% could not give any explanation or clarification of this term. As presented in Fig. 15, education is a dependent variable in this context. The higher the education, the better the knowledge regarding the concepts of 'Five Phases', 'Six Evils' and 'Seven Emotions'.

Furthermore, I must interpose a specific observation result here. Regarding the knowledge of certain Chinese medical concepts, I recognized a special interest in Chinese medicine among younger interviewees. The youngest age group (20-29 years) almost always achieves the highest rates in the self-reported familiarity with the medical concepts described above. Although these differences in data are not that striking at a first glance, the responses of younger participants were gradually more specific and more elaborate. Whereas people in their 40s or 50s very often only hesitantly answered my questions and pointed to other people around us because they thought that these people could make more specific statements regarding Chinese medicine; younger survey participants were clearly more confident about their knowledge regarding Chinese medicine. I further analyse this age-specific differentiation in the discussion and interpretation of the data.

As a last question regarding knowledge, I asked about the familiarity with the term 'psychotherapy' (*jingshen liaofa* 精神疗法). In contrast to the other terms named above, this phrase is taken from a biomedical paradigm and is not genuine to Chinese medicine. Nevertheless, whereas 35% of my informants reported that they do not know this term, 25% answered that they know it and 40% reported that they have at least heard of it. Among younger participants, the knowledge of 'psychotherapy' is above average with 73% of the 20-29 year old report to be familiar with it while among the oldest participants in contrast, 50% have never heard of this term before (Fig. 19).

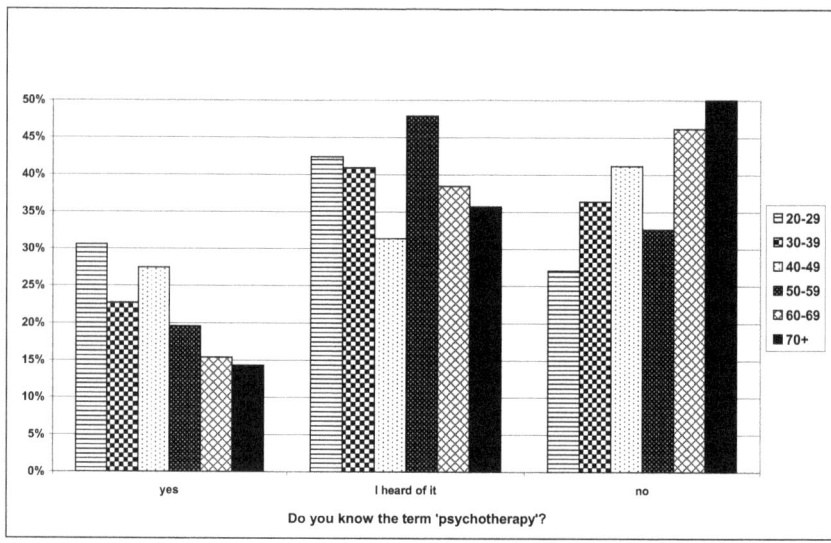

Fig. 19: *Self-reported knowledge of 'psychotherapy' (jingshen liaofa* 精神疗法*) according to age groups (Böke: Fieldwork 2010/2011).*

Younger urban inhabitants seem to have both a better knowledge of Chinese medicine and a better recognition of the Western medical term 'psychotherapy'. Looking closer into the reported meaning of the term 'psychotherapy' (*jingshen liaofa* 精神疗法), one finds a broad range of explanations, starting from a translation and transformation of this specific Western term 'psychotherapy' into a more genuine Chinese medical paradigm, *xinlixue* (心理学), to the more Western-influenced description of a 'conversational therapy' (*shuohua liaotian de zhiliaofa* 说话聊天的治疗法). A few interviewees related the treatment of insomnia (*zhiliao shuimian bu hao de ren*治疗睡眠不好的人) to this method, whereas others emphasized the 'stress-releasing function' (*huanjie yali de fangfa* 缓解压力的方法) of this therapy (Fig 20).

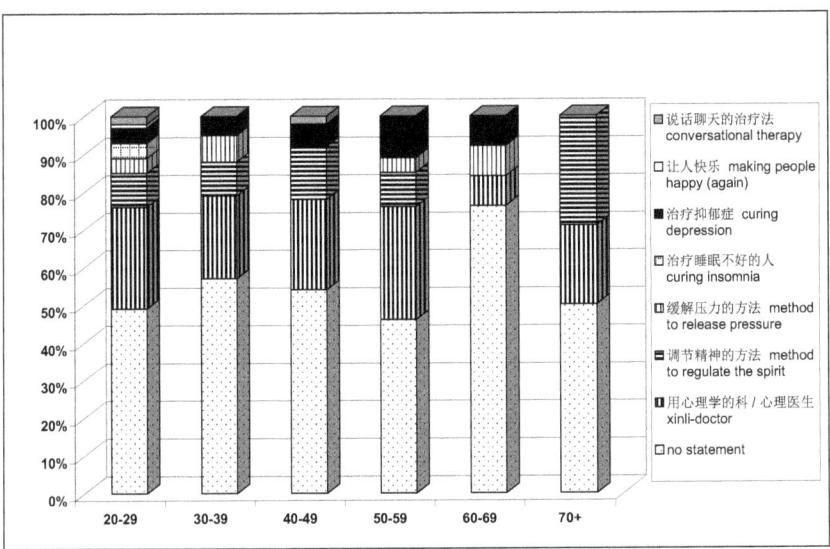

Fig. 20: Perceived meaning of the term 'psychotherapy' (jingshen liaofa 精神疗法) according to age groups (Böke: Fieldwork 2010/2011).

Although approximately 65% of the survey participants reported that they had at least heard of the term 'psychotherapy' (*jingshen liaofa* 精神疗法), it is obvious that in actuality, only a minority is indeed familiar with this term. However, the broadest range of explanations again was given by the youngest age group.

As will be shown in the discussion of the survey results, Chinese doctors report that especially the younger generations are very keen to preserve their health, in particular in regard to their status of emotional health. This coincides with the findings of the survey; younger people tend to name more 'psyche-related' diseases as caused by emotions, are more familiar with Chinese medical concepts such as the 'Seven Emotions' and are more acquainted to Western counselling methods such as 'psychotherapy'.

Sources of Knowledge

The self-reported sources of medical knowledge for the Beijing urban population are manifold. They range from written media such as books and magazines to conversations with family members, friends and doctors to internet resources.

However, the main source is infotainment television shows with Chinese medical content, and this outnumbers the other sources significantly (Fig. 21).

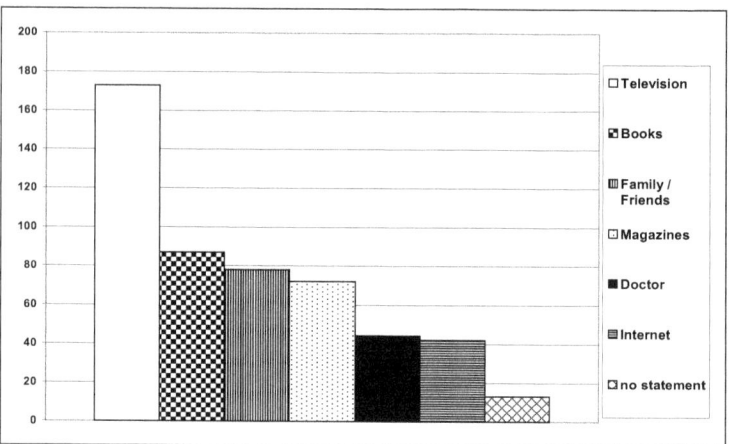

Fig. 21: *Sources of medical knowledge (total numbers of indications of 253 interviewees, multiple entries possible) (Böke: Fieldwork 2010/2011).*

Television was indicated 173 times, which means that almost 68% of all survey participants (n=253) named television as a source of their medical knowledge. As multiple answers were permitted, books were listed on 34% of all questionnaires, family and friends as sources were listed by 31% of the interviewees, and magazines covered 28% of the answers. The sources doctor and internet were only listed by 17% and 16% of the survey participants respectively. The television shows are equally popular among women and men, old and young, richer and poorer and educated and uneducated alike.

The prominent role of television in shaping the ideas of the population concerning Chinese medicine are perceived as ambivalent by professionals of Chinese medicine (as discussed in subchapter 6.2.2). On the one hand, they emphasize that this is a good way of spreading knowledge to the general public; on the other hand, they criticize oversimplification of Chinese medical theory and practice and the impression supported by these television shows that Chinese medicine can work miracle healing.

Different Medical Systems in Beijing

Up to now I presented data according to self-reported information about general evaluations of health and illness and about knowledge of certain concepts of Chinese medicine. To gain more insight into concrete practice, I furthermore asked the survey participants about the availability of different medical systems in Beijing and about their usage of these different medical systems in the last year. The additional question about the illnesses which were responsible for this usage was clearly marked optional due to ethical considerations, as I did not want to hurt my interviewee's privacy and prevent embarrassment and resistance. Consequently, only a deminishing minority responded to this question.

Not very surprising, every survey participant listed Chinese and Western medicine to be available in Beijing. However, with regard to other medical systems attributed to different ethnic minorities such as Tibetan, Mongolian or Miao, there was no consensus about the existence and availability of these medical systems in the capital. Whereas 21% of the 253 participants reported that beside Chinese and Western medicine, Tibetan medicine is available, more medical systems attributed to other ethnic groups were reported only in small amount (Fig. 22). Other 'foreign' medical concepts beside Western medicine, for example Ayurveda, Unani or Homeopathy, were not listed at all by the interviewees, although it can be assumed that at least some of these medical systems are present in Beijing. I can only speculate that these 'foreign' medical systems are not relevant for common urban dweller's daily medical practices and are maybe not perceived to be an essential part of Beijing's healthcare system.

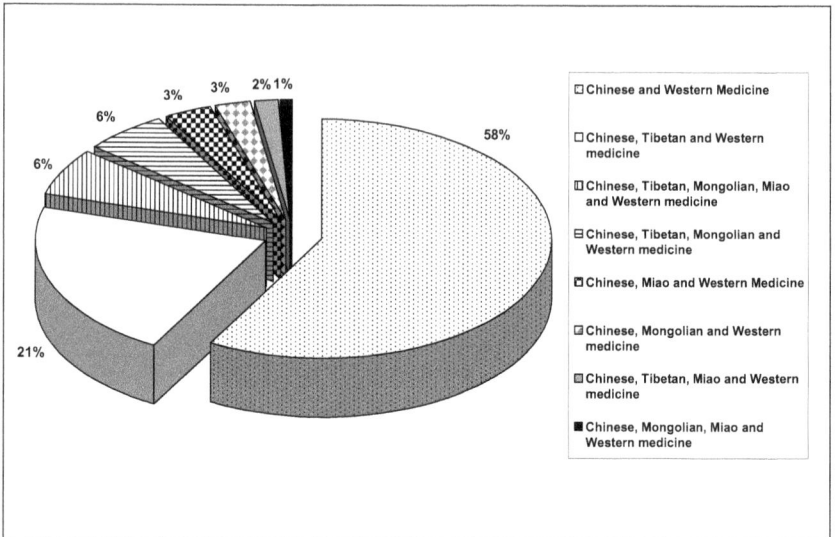

Fig. 22: Perceived availability of different medical systems in Beijing (Böke: Fieldwork 2010/2011).

Investigating the answers regarding the actual consultation of different medical systems during the last year, one finds a slight preponderance of Western medicine (Fig. 23), although many interviewees had no medical examination in the last year. Actually, more than half of the 253 respondents did not visit a doctor in the last year at all, whereas 21 % relied on Western medicine alone, 13 % made use of both the Western and Chinese medical system and only 12 % relied exclusively on the Chinese medical system. Medical systems attributed to ethnic minorities ('Mongolian' *meng*蒙 , 'Miao' *miao*苗 and 'Tibetan' *zang*藏) were only listed by single individuals, which is surprising because ethnic minorities' medicine is promoted strongly in newspapers, magazines and advertisement, and as Fig. 22 shows, is according to the informants, at least partially perceived available in Beijing.

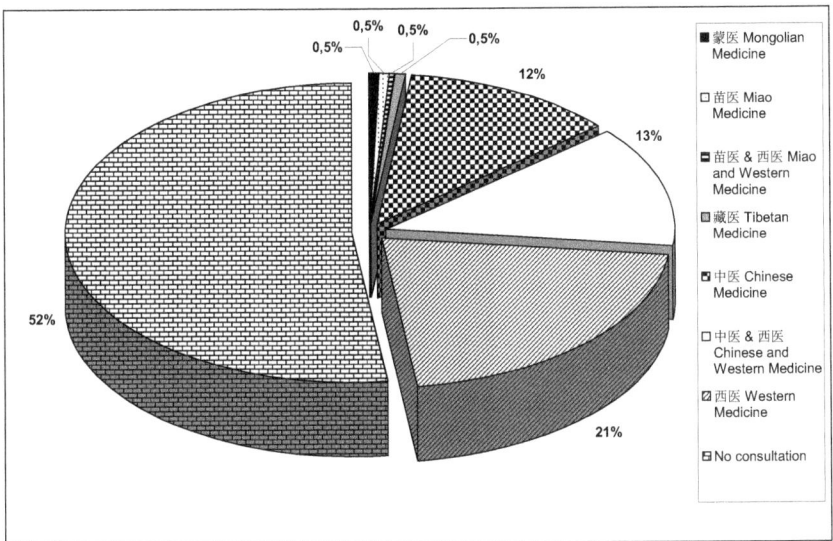

Fig. 23: Reported consultation of different medical systems in the last year (Böke: Fieldwork 2010/2011).

The reported usage of the different medical systems clearly presents patterns related to educational and economical background of the interviewees. There is a positive correlation between higher education and higher income on the one side, and a higher reliance to Chinese medicine on the other. University-graduates reported more than average that they solely used Chinese medicine in the last year. Among holders of Masters-degrees, 21 % reported that they solely consulted Chinese doctors; among holders of Bachelor-degrees 29 % also did so. In contrast, among people with middle school qualification, only six percent relied on Chinese medicine alone. Among people with only primary school qualification, nobody reported the exclusive usage of the Chinese medical system. Contrary, in these two last groups, almost half of the interviewees reported that they solely relied on Western medicine in the last year.

The relationship between income and usage of medical systems in the self reports of the informants reveals a similar pattern of correlation. Two-thirds of the lower income group[107] used Western medicine instead of Chinese medicine

---

107   The survey participant's income is scaled into six groups according to monthly income: less than 1000¥ RMB, 1000-2000¥ RMB, 2000-3000¥ RMB, 3000-4000¥ RMB, 4000-5000¥ RMB, more than 5000¥ RMB. According to the Statistical Yearbook 2010 by the Chinese government, the average per capita annual disposable income of urban house-

during the last year; in higher income groups this ratio is almost balanced. It can be expected that these education-specific and economical-specific answering patterns are at least partially evoked by the same set of survey participants, as a higher education commonly creates the opportunity to achieve a better income. These results are discussed in more detail in subchapter 6.1.4.4., because they are contrary to common estimations of Chinese medicine as being especially attractive to people with lower incomes.

Additionally, the reported usage of the different medical systems also presents patterns related to gender (Fig. 24 and 25). Male and female respondents reported almost equally about their consultation of Chinese medicine (male 13%, female 12%) and Western medicine (male 20%, female 21%) during the last year, but the combined consultation of both medical institutions in one year seems to be, as data reveals, a rather female-specific phenomenon (male 7%, female 19%).

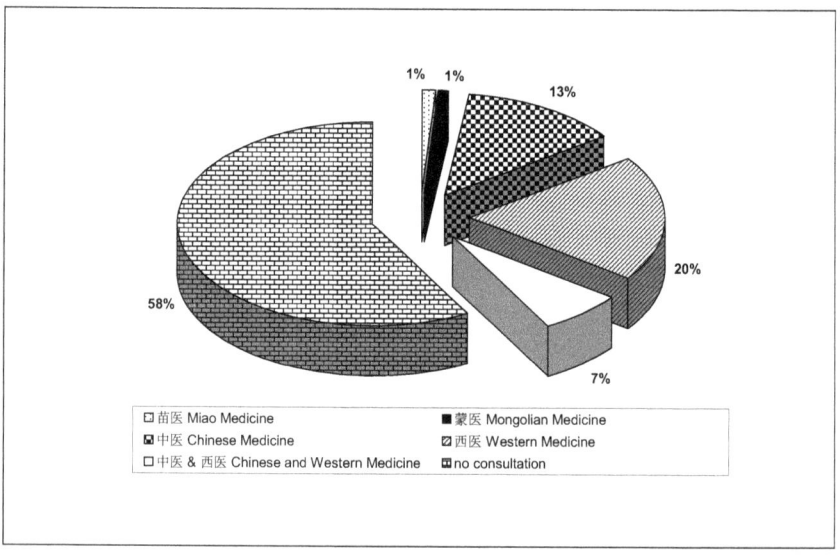

Fig. 24: *Reported consultation of different medical systems in the last year by men (Böke: Fieldwork 2010/2011).*

holds is 17.174,7¥ RMB (National Bureau of Statistics of China (2011): China Statistical Yearbook 2010. http://www.stats.gov.cn/tjsj/ndsj/2010/ html/ J1002c.htm ; last accessed at 16.11.2011)

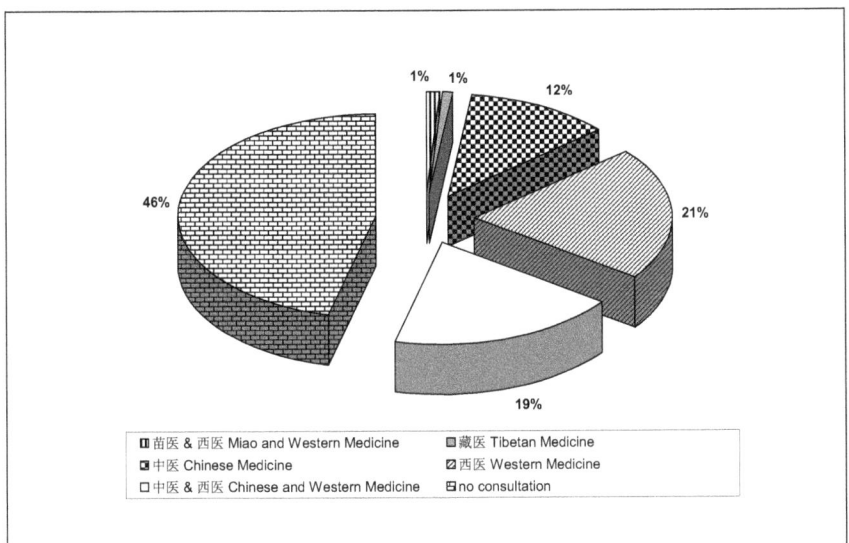

Fig. 25: Reported consultations of different medical systems in the last year by women (Böke: Fieldwork 2010/2011).

As will be discussed later on, this coincides with women's perspective and evaluation of Western gynaecology and Chinese concepts on women's medicine.

'Measuring' Urban Chinese Inhabitants' Attitudes on Chinese Medicine

In addition to the already presented dichotomous, polytomous and open answers revealing urban Chinese inhabitant's self reported view on Chinese medicine, I used a statistical method to 'measure' their attitudes on Chinese medicine and on perceived pathologic potential of emotions by using a 'Likert-Scale'.

The Likert-Scale[108] (named after Rensis Likert, 1903-1981, see Likert 1931) is a statistical tool used to explore and visualize people's attitudes toward specific topics in a bipolar scale ranging from total rejection to total acceptance. As

---

108 For a more detailed description of this method see Diekmann 2009: 240-270.

114

already explained above, I asked the questionnaire survey participants to either accept or reject statements concerning Chinese medicine in general and concerning the relationship between emotions and health in detail. The interviewees were requested to rate these statements on a scale from one (total rejection) to five (total acceptance).

General Attitudes on Chinese Medicine

I constructed five statements which should provide information about the general attitudes on Chinese medicine. These statements in particular were as follows:

1. Chinese medicine is better than Western medicine,
2. The "Six Evils" is an important pathological category,
3. The "Seven Emotions" is an important pathological category[109],
4. Western medicine is more scientific than Chinese medicine, and
5. Western medicine is more modern than Chinese medicine.

For evaluation, the results of the both last items had to be commutated. As already explained, the informants had to rate these statements on a scale from one (total rejection) to five (total acceptance) crossing three (undecided). Having five items, hypothetically an individual totally supporting Chinese medicine could score a sum of 25, while an also hypothetic individual totally rejecting Chinese medicine would only score a sum of five.

To determine whether these items indeed measure the targeted attitudes, I computed the so called correlation or discriminatory coefficient. The correlation coefficient of the last four items is comparatively high with values between 0.45 and 0.66 respectively. Only the first item, the direct statement that Chinese medicine is better than Western medicine, achieved a comparatively low correlation

---

109 One may object that the statements regarding the ‚Six Evils' and the ‚Seven Emotions' are confusing or pointing into a different direction, because the informants as shown in the preceding paragraphs are not aware of the specific meaning of these concepts. But I think, here one has to keep in mind the chronology of the questionnaire. As these statements were localized after the questions directly touching these concepts, the participants at that time were fully aware that 'Six Evils' and 'Seven Emotions' are indigenous medical concepts. Therefore I think it is justified to use these items as markers showing the attitudes towards Chinese medicine.

coefficient of only 0.34. Although Diekmann (2009: 246) ironically comments that a value of 0.40 or below is "not a phenomenal high value", I nevertheless decided to include this item because of the clear formulation of the statement. Accordingly, the average correlation coefficient of these five items still is 0.51, which is a proper and reliable value. To prove the internal reliability of these items building the backbone of the Likert-scale, I tested them with the statistical procedure 'Cronbach's alpha' (see Cronbach 1951), which gives a value for internal consistency. As George and Mallery (2002: 231) show, a Cronbach's alpha of $\alpha > 0.7$ is acceptable, $\alpha > 0.8$ is good and $\alpha > 0.9$ is excellent for sociological data sets. For this particular scale describing urban Chinese inhabitants attitude on Chinese medicine one can compute an alpha of $\alpha = 0.83$.

In total I evaluated 252 questionnaires for this analysis. The data reveals that the highest actual sum-score is 23 (25 would be the hypothetic maximum), while the lowest score actually is nine (five would be the hypothetic minimum). The first quartile (Q1) is at 15, which means that 25 % of the sum-scores of all interviewees are between 9 and 15. The second quartile, the median[110], is at 16. The third quartile is at 17, which means that 25 % of the sum-scores are between 17 and 22.

In transforming the collected data into a graph, one sees a more or less typical bell curve (*Gauß*-distribution) (Fig. 26) with a peak at the modus[111] of 15.

---

110 On an ordinal scale like the Likert-scale, the median separates the sample exactly in the middle.
111 The modus is the most often detected value in a data set.

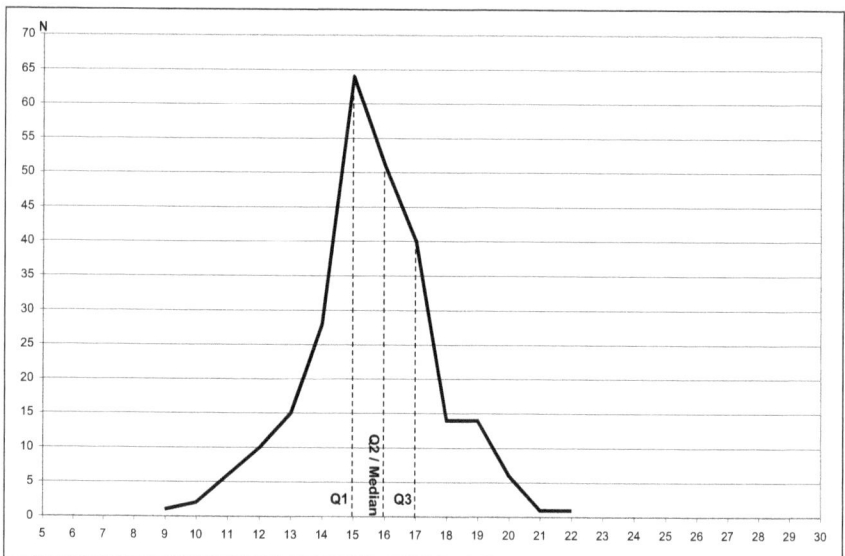

Fig. 26: Attitudes on Chinese medicine: distribution of sum-scores (Böke: Fieldwork 2010/2011).

One can see that Chinese urban inhabitants in general are somehow reluctant in their attitudes towards Chinese medicine. The hypothetical sum-score one would obtain if only choosing option three ('undecided') is 15. In this specific data set, this score coincides with the modus. The median is only gradually shifted to the right, showing that only a very tenuous majority of interviewees obtained higher-than-average sum-scores. This means that Chinese urban inhabitant's attitudes on Chinese medicine are more or less balanced and only a narrow majority approves Chinese medicine.

If one itemizes this scale into age cohorts, one finds a rather congruent distribution pattern (Fig. 27). The medians (Q2) of the age cohorts are disseminated only gradually, ranging from 15 for the youngest cohorts (20-29 years) to 16 for the mid-aged (40-49) to 17 for the oldest group (60 and older).

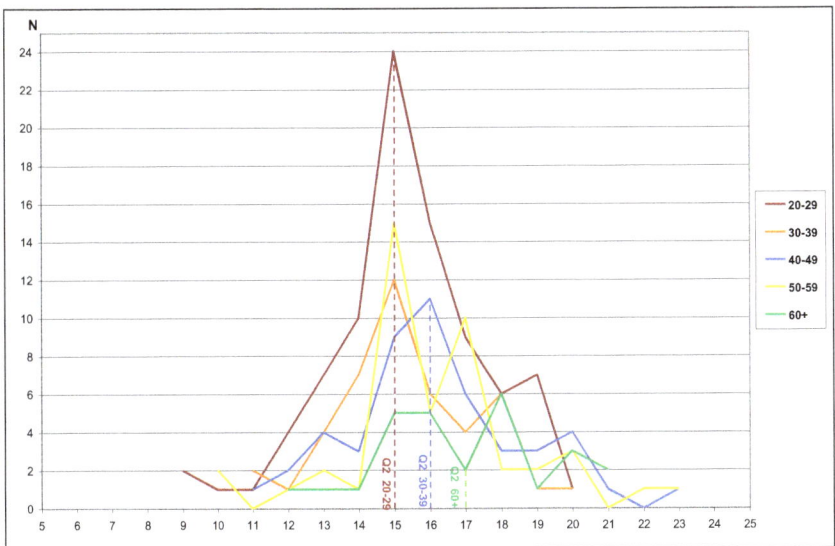

Fig. 27: Attitudes on Chinese medicine: distribution of sum-scores according to age (Böke: Fieldwork 2010/2011).

The peaks are all gathered in the medium range with a slight shift to the right and a second, considerably smaller peak on the right. One may speculate that this imbalance on the right side, especially visible in older age cohorts, might illustrate a higher regard for Chinese medicine in these particular age groups. However, in my opinion this interpretation would be debatable because it is clearly contrary to other observations as I will expose later on.

Regarding gender, one cannot find any obvious differences and the graphs of the Likert Scale are more or less parallel (Fig. 28). One can notice a slight shift of the median (Q2) from a sum-score of 15 (male) to 16 (female), but this is supposedly without statistical significance.

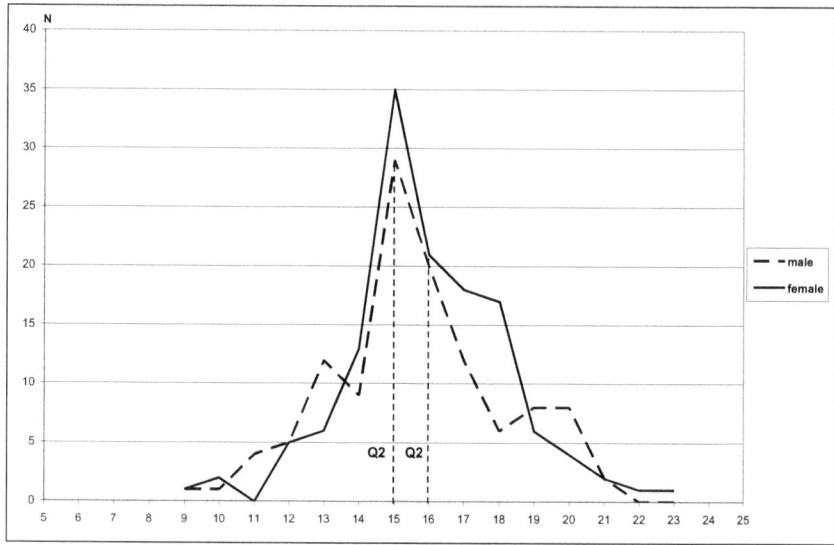

Fig. 28: Attitudes on Chinese medicine: distribution of sum-scores according to gender
(Böke: Fieldwork 2010/2011).

Accordingly, there seems to be no significant gender-difference concerning the general appraisement of Chinese medicine. The same is true for other evaluation dimensions applied in this study such as economic status and educational background. Analysing these dimensions, one does not perceive any relevant peculiarities.

Estimating the Pathological Potential of Emotions

Applying the same statistical tool to the question of how Chinese urban inhabitants estimate the pathological potential of emotions, I constructed seven statements which had to be approved or rejected by my informants. In detail, these statements are the following:

1. Emotions can influence health,
2. Emotional problems can lead to illnesses,

3. Chinese medicine tries to cure illnesses related to emotions,
4. Emotions can influence illnesses,
5. Emotions do not have influence on health,
6. Emotional excess can be harmful for the body, and
7. Emotions can harm 'organs' (*zangfu* 臟腑).

Again my informants had to rate these statements by ticking numbers from one (total rejection) to five (total acceptance) crossing three (undecided). During evaluation, item five had to be commutated. Having seven items, a hypothetical individual totally accepting these statements could score a sum of 35, while an also hypothetical individual totally rejecting the statements would only score a sum of seven.

To warrant applicability, I again computed the correlation coefficient for all statements. Statement six achieves a lower correlation coefficient of 0.4, while the values for the other statements are all between 0.5 and 0.8, revealing an average correlation coefficient of 0.7. Furthermore, I again computed the 'Cronbach's alpha' to prove internal consistency. Here I reach a very high value of $\alpha = 0.9$, which means that internal consistency here is beyond doubt.

This sample is composed of 252 questionnaires. The maximum sum-score of 35 is reached by 18 individuals while the lowest sum-score of 15 (seven would be the hypothetical minimum sum) is reached by two. The first quartile (Q1) is at 24, which means that a quarter of the interviewees scored sums between 15 and 24. The second quartile (Q2), the median, is at 27, while the third quartile (Q3) is at 31. Consequently, 25 % of the interviewees scored sums between 31 and the maximum of 35. The modus is at 25. Looking closer at the graph constructed out of this data, one finds a very asymmetric distribution of the sum-scores to the right side of the table (Fig. 29).

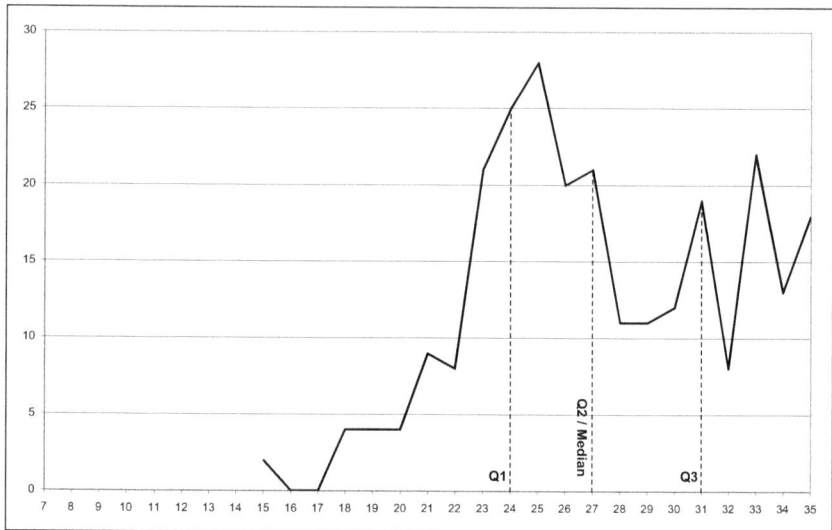

Fig. 29: *Attitudes on pathological potential of emotions: distribution of sum-scores (Böke: Fieldwork 2010/2011).*

This distribution discloses that a very high number of survey participants accepted the assertions of the presented statements. In a Gauß-distribution, one would expect the median around 21, which is the sum-score one would hypothetically achieve by only choosing the option 'undecided' (option number three). However, here more than 75 % of all sum-scores exceed 21 and the median is at 27, which already denotes a strong value of approval of the statements, meaning a strong support of assertions predicate the effect of emotions on human health.

A subdivision of this sample into different educational levels reveals a remarkable pattern. I combined people holding a Masters (MA) or Bachelors (BA) degree into subgroup 'higher formal education' (42 individuals), people with middle or primary school education are clustered under the label 'lower formal education' (35 individuals), whereas people with a distinct technical orientation in education (for example graduates of technical institutions) are grouped under 'technical education' (62 individuals). As Fig. 30 demonstrates, people with technical orientation score significantly lower sum-scores than the other two groups. The median (Q2) in this group is at 24, which mean that also among the technically focused urban population, the concept of emotions as pathogenic agents is prevailing, but only reluctantly. In contrast, looking at university graduates holding a Master or Bachelor degree, the median (Q2) is shifted to 26. People clustered in this group score higher sum-scores because they tend to accept statements claiming the pathological potential of emotions more firmly, but the graph shows a higher variety of estimations as it has not just one paramount peak but a broader distribution. The highest sum-scores though is obtained by people with lower education. Here the median (Q2) is at 29, which means that 50 % scored higher sum-scores, a value clearly beyond average.

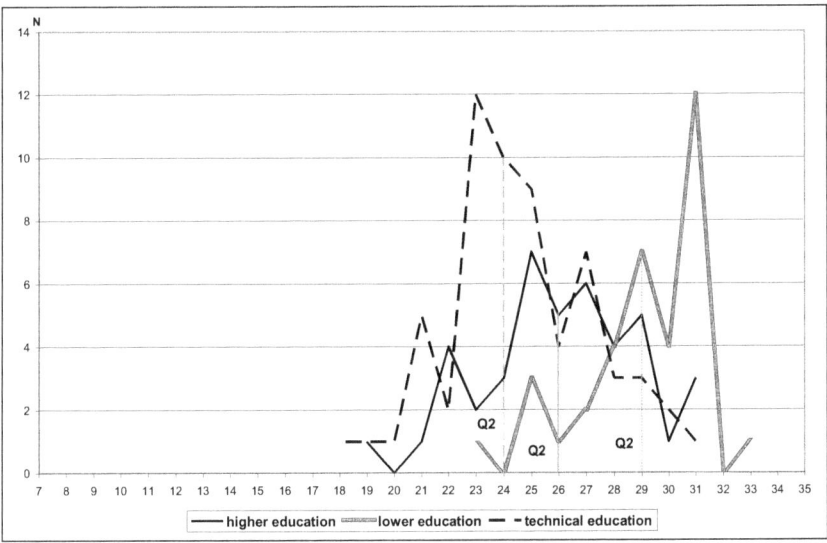

Fig. 30: *Attitudes on pathological potential of emotions: distribution of sum-scores according to educational background (Böke: Fieldwork 2010/2011).*

Obviously there is a stronger tendency among lower educated people to emphasize the pathological quality of emotions, together with a significant conformity, whereas among the higher educated group the range of dispersion is more extensive. People with technical education background tend to focus more on the biomedical explanation schemes concerning illnesses as opposed to the pathologic consequences of emotions.

Discussion

In the following subchapters I discuss the survey results in broader categories of appraisal and status of Chinese medicine in Beijing society. Thereby I focus on the familiarity with Chinese medical concepts and the general evaluation of Chinese medicine, on the perceived pathological potential of emotions and on group-specific perceptions of illnesses caused by emotions as well as on the utilization of Chinese medicine.

Beijing Inhabitants' Familiarity with Chinese Medical Concepts and the Evaluation of Chinese Medicine

As shown in the statistical analysis, I inquired after three main concepts of Chinese medicine, the 'Five Phases', the 'Six Evils' and the 'Seven Emotions' to establish knowledge. Furthermore, I asked about a prominent classical book on Chinese medicine, the *Huangdi neijing*. The responses to these questions were quite diverging. While, for example the concept of the 'Seven Emotions' was fairly well-known and also a majority of participants claimed that they at least had heard of the book *Huangdi neijing*, the majority of interviewees were rather unacquainted with the concepts of the 'Five Phases' and especially with the 'Six Evils'.

A high proportion of middle aged and older people almost reflexively repelled my request to take part in the survey and pointed to bystanders, which in their view could offer a broader knowledge of Chinese medicine. Even if I consider that sometimes this behaviour surely works as an excuse to refuse the participation in the survey, it reveals that a considerable amount of middle aged people evaluated their own knowledge on Chinese medicine as insufficient and were only hesitantly willing to unveil it. However, this behaviour was quite atypical for younger survey participants (20-29 years old). This cohort normally openly answered the questions, showed no hesitance but conveyed a sense of confidence. These young people seemed to be very interested in Chinese medical concepts and often reported that they are fond of therapies rooted in Chinese medicine, especially naming acupuncture. As will be shown in Chapter 6, this view is also shared by Chinese medical professionals, who certified that the younger generation is especially interested in Chinese medicine and they are common visitors of Chinese medical clinics.

Infotainment television shows are to a high degree (see Fig. 21) responsible for the imparting of knowledge of Chinese medicine. It is the most common source for Beijing inhabitants and its prevalence is not a matter of age, education or gender. After books, family and friends and magazines, conversation with doctors is only a subordinate source and some informants told me that Chinese doctors only ask but do not explain. However, this is somehow contradictory to findings I present in expert interviews, where repeatedly was stated that the explanation of disease mechanisms is an important part of therapy.

With regard to the general evaluation of Chinese medicine, especially in contrast to Western biomedicine, I collected several informal statements expressed by the survey participants. They commonly emphasized that 'Chinese medicine works slowly, whereas Western medicine works quickly' (*zhongyi man xiyi kuai* 中医慢西医快)[112]. However, only a few people regarded this as an advantage of Western medicine ('Western medicine is quick and simple, Chinese medicine is slow and inconvenient' *xiyi kuai he jiandan, zhongyi man he bu fangbian* 西医快和简单，中医慢和不方便). Most of the informants connected the 'slowness' of Chinese medicine with a deeper and more careful functioning, frequently stating that 'Western medicine works fast, but does not treat the root, whereas Chinese medicine works slow, but does treat the root' (*xiyi haode kuai, bu yi de gen. Zhongyi haode man, yi de gen* 西医好得快，不医的根。中医好得慢，医的根). Others branded Western medicine as 'focusing on superficial phenomena, whereas Chinese medicine focuses on the true source of the ailment' (*xiyi zhenliao biao, zhongyi zhenliao ben* 西医诊疗表，中医诊疗本). However, only a minority expressed their refusal of Western medicine because of the 'high amount of side-effects' (*fuzuoyong tai da le* 副作用太大了). The vast majority of informants stated very pragmatically that 'both medical systems, the Chinese and the Western, had their own advantages' (*ge you ge hao* 各有个好). Furthermore, a few people stated that the focus should be on the specific doctor rather than on the medical system, because doctors are not equally good (*daifu ye bu tong* 大夫也不同). From this perspective, the quality of the doctor and not its affiliation to a specific medical system is the relevant point for people's evaluation. Additionally, it was commonly agreed on that both Chinese and Western medicine have medical specialities (*zhongxiyi ge you techang* 中西医各有特长).

---

112 The Chinese phrases in the brackets are quotations from my interviews. I paraphrased these quotations in the English text.

The Pathological Potential of Emotions

In contrast to the familiarity with Chinese medical concepts, the evaluation of the pathologic potential of emotions united a sweeping majority of study participants. People not only strongly affirmed questions pertaining to whether emotions can cause illnesses ('of course they can' *dangran keyi* 当然可以), but additionally emphasized their answers with nodding approval. Regarding this topic, many people reacted openly and equipped me with further data by making additional statements. A common assertion was that all emotions can do harm when in excess (*guodule dou bu hao* 过渡了都不好). Also in these informal conversations, I observed a tendency to particularly emphasize the pathologic potential of anger. One informant generally condemned anger and expressed that human should fear anger (*ren gai pa shengqi* 人该怕生气) because of its pathologic potential. A majority of informants stated that anger can influence every organ or harm the whole body (*shengqi dui shenti bu hao* 生气对身体不好). Furthermore, I collected statements totally in line with assertions in ancient classics and modern textbooks, namely that anger especially harms the liver (*nu shang gan* 怒伤肝).

Anger is quite a significant emotion because it intimately refers to social stability. This social stability is endangered, if one follows Berkowitz and Harmon-Jones (2004) in their definition of anger as "a syndrome of relatively specific feelings, cognitions and physiological reactions *linked associatively with an urge to injure some target*" (Berkowitz & Harmon-Jones 2004: 108, emphasis added). In a society like the Chinese, where social harmony is not only a shared value introduced by philosophy several thousand years ago, but is also instrumented in recent political thought and slogan (for example the 'Harmonious Society' *hexie shehui* 和谐社会[113]). Anger and its deeply disturbing potential for violent outbreak, is therefore consequently regarded as very dangerous, on the macro-level (on political level) as well as on the micro-level (the individual body). Bond (1993) outlines the connection between a healthy body and a healthy social environment in detail:

> [...] the goal is maintaining emotional balance to protect internal homeostasis. Chinese cosmology and phenomenology draw no distinction between forces internal

---

113 This concept was introduced by Chinese President Hu Jintao after his succession to power in 2002 as a guideline for his administration in political, economical, cultural and environmental issues. It was also incorporated into into the Chinese government's 11th five-year plan (2006–2010). For further information see Lam 2005 and Delury 2008.

and external to the body, so that social interchanges must be carefully monitored and managed in order to guard one's internal condition. Considerable attention is paid to maintaining a state of interpersonal harmony in one's social network. Hostile behaviour, in particular, is avoided, [...] caution in speech is constantly encouraged, [...] interpersonal problems are presented in less threatening symptomology (Bond 1993: 256).

My informants regarded anger as the most dangerous emotion for individual and (one may add) societal health.

Furthermore, a common issue came up on which the questionnaire had not focussed on, i.e. the connection between emotions, ingestion and health.[114] Routinely people described that emotional instability can lead to a lack of appetite which weakens the body and leads to illnesses. A common formulation was that "when the emotions are not well [meaning not appropriately balanced], one refuses to eat" (*qingxu bu hao chifan bu xiang chi* 情绪不好吃饭不想吃) or one develops a "lack of appetite" (*shiyu bu hao* 食欲不好). Therefore, many people regarded the stomach as being easily endangered by emotions (*qingzhi dui wei weixian* 情志对胃危险).

If one compares the lists of potentially pathologic emotions given by informants and the lists of emotion terms perceived by the informants as being part of the concept of 'Seven Emotions' (Fig. 19), one finds two striking characteristics. The list enumerating the 'Seven Emotions' both show significantly lower diversity and a different composition of emotional terms as opposed to the free list generated by participants of potentially pathologic emotions. This means that the Beijing urban population considers many more emotions to be pathologic than just those belonging to the category of the 'Seven Emotions'. One furthermore can estimate a discrepancy between theory and practice. For example, the theoretically potential pathogenic emotions 'happiness' (*xi* 喜) or 'joy' (*le* 乐), although commonly identified by the survey participants as belonging to the 'Seven Emotions', are not often named as causing illnesses in the question regarding

---

114 Some scholars like Anderson (1990: x) attested Chinese society a "fascination with food", while a famous, paradigmatic Chinese novel, "The Gourmet" (meishijia 美食家) by Lu Wenfu (陆文夫), organizes its storyline along this topic. For an ethnological overview about food in modern China see Farquhar 2002:1-166. Chinese cookbooks routinely refer to the medical quality of the described meal. For the relevance of regulated ingestion of suitable food for Chinese medicine also see Farquhar 1994b.

the pathologic potential of emotions. On the other hand, while 'anger' (at least represented in the more colloquial term *shengqi* 生气) is the most commonly listed illness inducing emotion; only seven interviewees attribute this term to the 'Seven Emotions'.[115]

The emotions 'stress' (*jinzhang* 紧张) and 'pressure' (*yali* 压力) only perform a minor role in the statistical data evaluation, because they are named only a few times by young people.[116] However, especially young and well-educated survey participants frequently stated that 'pressure' and 'stress' are emotional conditions which they have to face and which can easily lead to illnesses. One statement of a 24 year old woman interviewed in *Haidian* District (海淀区), who reported an episode where her husband suffered from 'pressure', is paradigmatic:

> After our marriage, my husband came to town with me. But here he soon felt under pressure (*yali* 压力). This was due to the urban lifestyle, where everything is so fast and noisy. And he had problems at work, there he was under pressure, too, had to work extra hours. He became sick, so he returned to the countryside for a while and there he recovered.

Reports like this, although not always that specific, were disclosed frequently during my fieldwork. Beside the topic of 'work', which was important in the quotation above and in several other reports, the two additionally important factors 'family' and 'education' were mentioned as creating stress or pressure for young urban Chinese. The three terms collected in the survey expressing 'stress'

---

115   Although one could argue that this is subsumed in the term nu 怒 which is more common in written language and which is therefore the standard term for anger in Chinese medical theory. However, both terms are listed frequently as potentially pathogen emotions.

116   One may object that it has to be discussed whether stress or pressure are actually emotions. Because I rely on emic Chinese concepts of emotions, I avoid this discussion for three reasons. First, as terms meaning stress or pressure were noted in my questionnaire, I have to assume that this is a relevant emotional category for my informants. Second, while asking Chinese native speakers to cluster the emotion terms, they handled this category without hesitation as an emotion category, in explicit contrast to other terms like xiuse羞涩 (shyness) or jizao急躁 (irritableness), which they clustered as features of human character, not as emotions. And third, during interviews with Chinese medical experts, they also frequently referred to these terms and labelled them as emotions respectively labelled illnesses arising from stress and pressure as emotion-related.

or 'pressure' are *jinzhang* 紧张 , *yayi* 压抑and *yali*压力. The first term, *jinzhang* 紧张implies a concept more similar to the Western concept of 'stress', whereas the other two terms, *yayi* 压抑and *yali* 压力, share more similarity with the Western concept of 'being under pressure'.[117] I realized that most of my young and well-educated informants shared the idea of a three stage development, starting with stress leading to depression which finally culminated in more illnesses. This view is shared by medical experts, who also stated that stress and pressure are problems the urban youth has to deal with. Therefore I elaborate this topic more detailed in my analysis of the expert interviews in chapter 6.

Group-specific Perception of Illnesses Caused by Emotions

The statistical analysis of the empirical data collected reveals that, concerning the illnesses thought of as being caused by emotions, one can differentiate into two categories; namely 'somatic' illnesses (such as heart disease, liver disease etc.) and 'psychological' issues (such as depression, insanity etc.). Whereas the 'somatic' illnesses were stated by all groups of informants, no matter age, gender, education or economic status, the 'psychological' issues were mainly stated by specific participants, namely by a younger, well educated sub-sample (see Fig. 14b). Only one individual older than 60 named depression as an illness caused by emotions; in contrast, this was a common sentiment among younger participants. This tendency is also described by medical experts, as will be presented in chapter 6. It is not plausible that depression is not relevant for older people in China or that this specific group is less depressed than younger people. Indeed, research literature shows that depression, at least established according to Western biomedical standards, is also prevalent among older Chinese individuals (Phillips et al 2009, Chen et al. 2005).

Other explanatory models must be constructed. I think it is reasonable to focus on the different concepts behind depression, which the different interviewees might have. Depression is 'traditionally' stigmatized in Chinese culture. Re-

---

117 These terms do additionally carry the concrete meaning 'pressure' ya 压in a literal sense (for example xueya 血压blood pressure, or kongyaji 空压机compressor). This is not to confuse with the "container-under-pressure-metaphor" for anger, which can be found in several languages, among them German, English and Chinese (for example see Kövecses 1995, 1998; for Chinese especially see Yu 1995 and King 1989).

viewing the research literature on depression in China, one is inevitably confronted with an explanatory model called 'somatization' (see Chapter 5). Various studies, for example Kleinman's works (1979, 1982, 1986), show that Chinese patients usually tend to 'somatize', i.e. to primarily present 'somatic' symptoms while seeking 'psychological' help, and Lin et al. (1980: 253) indicate it as the "chief idiom through which Chinese culture articulates [...] neurotic disorders. Generally, 'somatization' is thought of as allowing individuals to inhabit the sick role. In certain societies, such as the Chinese, this role is socially more accepted than the stigmatized deviant role of the mental ill (Ryder et al. 2008: 302, c.f. Goldberg & Bridges 1988: 142-143). A consequence of this 'somatizing' behaviour is that during the patient-doctor-interaction in TCM, the direct reference to emotional states is avoided and the treatment is addressed primarily to somatic conditions (c.f. Wu 1982: 292), which further consolidates the stigmatization of emotional distress.

Emotional stability was for the most time of history a cultural imperative for Chinese society. Ots (1990: 25) identifies "a long standing tradition of repression of emotions [...] mainly based on Neo-Confucian ideals", whereas "emotional excess is highly stigmatized". Tung (1994: 488-490) emphasizes the Chinese self-conception as being "primarily social and interpersonal" and "concerned with constant judgement of one's being good or bad, right or wrong". When emotional equilibrium is a requested condition, emotional disorder, especially depression as a very strong state of disequilibrium, is a violation of this demand and offends the social context of the individual, as "one is fundamentally a part of a larger whole".

However, presumably there is a shift in the perceived stigmatizing potential of depression in different generations. Whereas older people still avoid talking about this topic, younger people are less inhibited. I think it is plausible to explain this shift with the specific historic experience older Chinese share. They experienced a period in Chinese history, where the expression of depression not only meant cultural and social stigma, but additionally and more dangerous and even life-threatening, entailed a political dimension. During political and economical tough times like the 'Great Leap Forward' (*da yue jin* 大跃进 1958-1961) or the 'Cultural Revolution' (*wenhua dageming* 文化大革命 1966-1976), the stigmatization of being emotionally instable was intensified. Emotional problems and especially depression were not only coded as endangering social harmony, but they were regarded as problems of the 'wrong political attitude', for a true and confident socialist or maoist could *per definitionem* not be distressed or depressed[118] (Chang et al. 2005:105, c.f. Parker et al. 2001:859). Mark Lupher (1999) describes the daily routine of political campaigns, mass movements and indoctrinations the youth and young adults of the 1950s and 1960s were exposed to; those that are in their 60s or 70s today. This ultimately culminated in the establishment of the 'Red Guards' (*hong weibing* 红卫兵), a paramilitary force of adolescents and young adults encouraging the Cultural Revolution (Fig. 31).

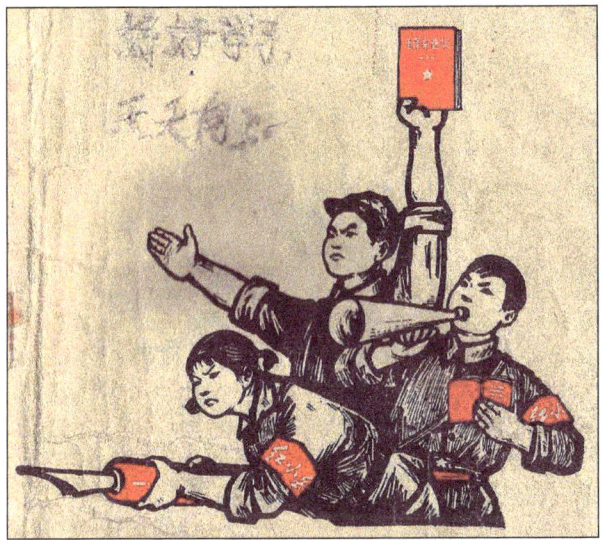

Fig. 31: *Young Red Guards on a cover of a 1971 schoolbook*[119]

Anita Chan (1985) also emphasizes the importance of maoist political indoctrination during socialization process of this "first generation brought up under socialism" (Chan 1985: 1) and Kleinman and Kleinman (1999:16-17) showed that traumatic events of these bygone period have consequences for the daily life

---

118 This is also true for other emotional spheres and practices. Pan & Huang (2011) show that other "passionate practices" like sexuality also contradicted with political targets of the Cultural Revolution and therefore were limited and regulated in order to avoid "any 'lifestyle problems' (shenghuo zuofeng 生活作风) or 'disordering of men and women's relationships' (luan gao nannü guanxi 乱搞男女关系) [which] were deemed a fatal threat" (222-223).

119 Source: Wikipedia, public domain (http://en.wikipedia.org/wiki/File:Red_Guards.jpg ; last access 28.09.2012).

some decades later, because in many cases there still is a social contact between 'victim' and 'committer' and therefore "deep feelings of anguish, anger, grief and revenge could not be worked trough"; as an informant of Arthur and Joan Kleinman explained:

> You try to forget it [the past], but how can you? You don't. They are here. And you are here. At night you dream of revenge. But by morning you have to get up and pass them in the streets (Kleinman and Kleinman 1999:17).

Consequently, many people are confronted with these times not only in their own personal history and experience, but also in daily social life. Medical experts also referred to this special experience of older people (see Chapter 6.2.4.).

However, to paraphrase a statement by Chan (1985: 225): The 2000s are not the 1950s; and the children of Hu Jintao are not the children of Mao Zedong. Therefore, the cultural as well as the political stigma, is much more degraded among the young urban inhabitants born in the 1980s and 1990s. Obviously, they did not experienced the times of the Great Leap Forward and the Cultural Revolution and escaped the political stigmatization of depression, and the impact of the cultural stigma of depression is lessened among younger Chinese through the flood of Western psychology and lifestyle. Ideas of depression and stress-related illnesses, not only as a clinical category, but as a consequence of a certain lifestyle which affects many people, are commonly spread in journals and magazines. Additionally, in chapter seven I will elaborate further reasons for the age-specific answers.

Utilization of Chinese Medicine

Educational and especially economic background seems to have influence on patient's choice of medical treatment, also contrary to common estimations on Chinese medicine. Whereas lower income groups are thought of visiting the Chinese medical system, commonly evaluated as comparatively inexpensive, instead of Western medical institutions, in my sample the lower income-groups had a two-third prevalence to use Western medicine instead of Chinese medicine, whereas in higher income groups this ratio is balanced. This view was expressed in informal conversations during the survey by many interviewees and also some of the professional doctors which I interviewed named Chinese medicine as especially attractive for patients with lower incomes. Despite this notion of Chinese medicine as being attractive for people with lower income, the relationship between better income and higher education on the one hand and a tendency to rely on the non-biomedical paradigm on the other, is similar to the usage of non-biomedical methods in Western societies. Research in Western societies reveals that, just like in this Chinese sample, users of non-biomedical treatment are more likely to have a high education, a rather prestigious occupation and are equipped with an above average household income (for example see Fox et al. 2010, Hunt et al. 2010, Barnes et al. 2008, Xue et al. 2007 or Barry 2005). Consequently, one can expect a similar set of explanation models for this chosen behaviour. The informal interviews among the survey participants reveal that people who choose Chinese medicine instead of Western medicine worried about the adverse effects of biomedicine and emphasized the inoffensiveness of Chinese medicine. Furthermore, they rejected Western medicine because they accused it of treating only the symptoms of the illness instead of its roots, a quality which they saw better implemented in Chinese medicine. Health is a common topic in the urban middle and upper-middle class and motives for choosing between different available medical systems are similar to motives of the same social groups in Western societies.

The data furthermore reveals a slight preference of Western medicine among women (see Fig. 25). In informal conversations, women told me that concerning "women's issues" they trust more in Western gynaecology than in Chinese women's medicine. This corresponds with conspicuous advertisement in Beijing. Especially on billboards in subway-stations or at crossroads, clinics exclusively devoted to women's health are advertised (Fig. 32.

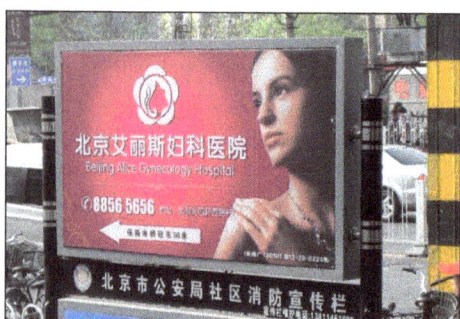 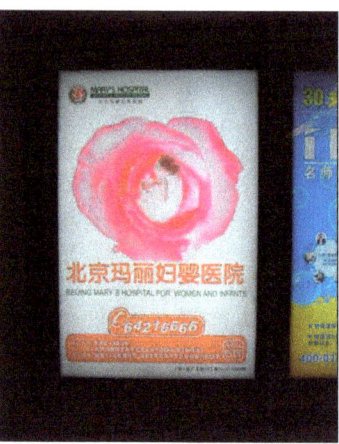

Fig. 32: Billboards advertising women's hospitals in Beijing (Böke: Fieldwork 2010/2011).

Concerning infant's medicine, I found a differentiated perception among my informants. Women emphasized that for prenatal, during birth and in early postnatal care, they trusted in Western medicine; after the early postnatal period, they also approved Chinese medicine, at least for specific illnesses. In this context it was usually stated that Chinese medicine had fewer side-effects than Western medicine and is therefore especially useful for breastfeeding mothers as well as more suitable for infants.

The Experts' Interviews

Aside from the survey questionnaire, I interviewed 20 experts of Chinese medicine, among them four students of Chinese medicine enrolled at the Beijing University of Chinese medicine (*Beijing Zhongyiyao Daxue*北京中医药大学), one clinic manager, three members of clinic staff and 12 doctors of Chinese medicine.[120] The clinics I visited were different in size and in objective. The first clinic, hereinafter called Clinic A, is a rather small sized outpatient clinic in the

---

120 For a description of these experts, see appendix 3. In the text I refer to the practitioners as 'doctors', using the translation of the Chinese title daifu 大夫 which is a honourable form of addressing for example people working as 'physician' or 'doctor', but does not denote the academic title (this would be boshi博士).

Haidian District, located at the edge of the extended city centre. According to self-description, this clinic focuses on outpatients with emotion- and stress-related disorders and mainly provides manual therapies like acupuncture with medical herbs only play a minor role. The second clinic (Clinic B) is a mid-size outpatient clinic focusing on broader public. The clinic manager explained the concept of providing the opportunity for common people to visit "famous doctors"; in this clinic doctors from important Chinese hospitals offer their services on specific days according to a schedule. Directly connected to this clinic is a pharmacy which sells Chinese ready-made drugs as well as individual drugs prepared according to doctor's prescription. Thirdly, I conducted research in one of the biggest Chinese hospitals in Beijing (Clinic C). This clinic offers a whole variety of treatments; for example, acupuncture, massage, Chinese as well as Western medical drugs and treatment were all available. Furthermore, it maintains a specialized department for insomnia patients. According to its own description, this institution spends annually up to 100 million RMB[121] for psychological research dealing with Chinese medical theory.

Except for the interviews with students, which were recorded at the campus of the Beijing University of Chinese Medicine and which took approximately 30 minutes each, all the other interviews were recorded in rooms of the respective institution employing the interview partners.[122] These interviews took approximately one hour. As I want to preserve the anonymity of my informants, their names have been replaced with aliases.[123]

The central questions in these semi-structured interviews can be clustered into four categories. First, I asked questions about the expert's view on the pathologic potential of emotions. The second category is build by questions regarding the consultations of patients and the estimation of their knowledge on emotions and their relevance for health. Third, I asked about the transfer of medical knowledge and the expert's opinion on TV infotainment shows with medical content. As a fourth point, I asked about patient's specific group behaviour (Table 3).

---

121 Approximately 10 million Euro.
122 With the exception of one student, all informants granted permission to be recorded on tape for the interviews. One interview was handwritten with the student who rejected this request. Two more interviews with practitioners were conducted spontaneously without the help of a tape recorder. These interviews were also handwritten.
123 Some of my informants explicitly demanded anonymity while others were not concerned of revealing their names. However, I decided to expose neither the identity of all my informants, nor the identity of the clinics.

Table 3: Question categories and exemplarily questions asked during the experts' interviews.

Category	Exemplarily questions
1. General questions about emotions and health	According to Chinese medicine, how are emotions and health connected? How do you typically treat illnesses caused by emotions?
2. Questions about patient's knowledge	Is Chinese medicine relevant for the population of Beijing? Do your patients know about the connection between emotions and illnesses?
3. Questions regarding knowledge transfer	How do you estimate the TV infotainment shows promoting Chinese medicine? What do you think of the growing relevance of Chinese medicine in Western societies?
4. Questions about group specific prevalence of certain illnesses	Do you see differences in coping with emotional problems among certain social groups? Are there certain social groups which are predominantly exposed to pathologic emotional experiences?

I did not use a strict guiding questionnaire with a binding sequence of questions but tried to be responsive and adjusted my questions to my interview partners. However, to enhance comparability, of course all broader question clusters were represented in the interviews.

Expert's View on Illness and Emotions

Understandably, all of the experts emphasized the pathologic potential of emotions. They all listed the 'Seven Emotions' according to standardized Chinese medical theory: 'happiness, anger, sorrow, excessive thinking, sadness, fear and fright' (xi, nu, you, si, bei, kong, jing 喜怒忧思悲恐惊). Doctor Li, a 27 year old junior practitioner working at Clinic A, explained paradigmatically the influence of emotions on bodily processes:

All emotions can be very harmful to the body (*qingzhi dui shenti dou hen wexian* 情志对身体都很危险). For example, if you get very angry, your blood pressure will immediately rise too high. If blood pressure is too high, this can be very dangerous to the blood vessels (*biru shuo, yi ge ren shengqi fanu de shihou ta de xueya jiu shi hen gao. Tebie gao de xueya hen weixian dui neizhong de xueguan* 比如说，一个人生气发怒的时候他的血压就是很高。特别高的血压很危险对内中的血管) (Interview with Dr. Li; Böke: Fieldwork 2010/2011).

Doctor Zhang, the mid-aged vice-director of this clinic, emphasized that emotions are internal causes (*limian de yinsu* 里面的因素, or *neiyin* 内因) for illness. These inner causes have more influence on the body than outer causes and emotions in general can harm the organs (*qingzhi shang zangfu* 情志伤脏腑). He furthermore explains that emotions influence the movement of *qi* 气: for example, anger makes *qi* rise high, fear makes *qi* sink down. As *qi* has, according to Chinese medical theory, the function to control the movement of blood (*qi kongzhi xue* 气控制血), during episodes of anger the blood rises simultaneously with the *qi*, whereas during episodes of fear, the blood sinks down. By this, he continued, the whole body is directly affected through emotional experience.

The 28 year old Doctor Liu explained that emotional instability is especially dangerous to patients who already have organic problems, a position which was supported by many other practitioners. In a case of pre-existing illness or weakening, primarily the five emotions happiness, anger, sadness, fear and fright may cause additional hardship (*wu zhong qingxu xi nu bei kong jing dou hui changsheng shanghai* 五种情绪喜怒悲恐惊都会产生伤害).

A more vivid description of the connection between emotions and illness was provided by a 59 year old staff member of a Chinese clinic. She reported the influence of emotions on her husband's health; on the one hand, she describes the connection between anger, liver and eyes, on the other hand she draws a connection between lungs and sadness:

> Emotions can have severe influence on human's health (*qingzhi dui ren de jiankang you jilie de guanxi* 情志对人的健康有激烈的关系). My husband use to get angry very quickly. As anger harms the liver (*nu shang gan* 怒伤肝), so he frequently has problems with his liver (*ta youshi you ganzang de chuwenti* 他有时有肝脏的出问题). Because the liver is connected to the eyes, his eyes are also easily worsens (*gan yingxiang mu, suoyi yanjing rongyi cha gan* 肝影响目，所以眼睛容易差 gan) (Interview with a female clinic staff member; Böke: Fieldwork 2010/2011).

She furthermore outlined that the organ corresponding to sadness is the lung and that therefore sadness can lead to lung problems (*youchou keyi zaocheng fei de chuwenti* 忧愁可以造成肺的出问题).

The statements of all practitioners are very similar: during interviews they all emphasize the pathologic effect of emotions, list the 'Seven Emotions' according to standardized Chinese medical theory and relate emotions to *qi* and blood. However, even among the practitioners there is a tendency to especially emphasize the pathological quality of anger and the susceptibility of the heart and the liver. The 24 year old junior practitioner Doctor Wang explained that anger rises up from the liver and manifests in the red face a person gets when he or she is angry. He referred to a Chinese idiomatic expression *nu fa chong guan* 怒发冲冠 which literally means that someone is so angry that his hair perks up and pushes away the hat to demonstrate the 'rising' characteristic of anger.[124] Doctor Sun, a 37 year old practitioner of Chinese medicine, regards some organs to be linked more close to emotions than others. He said that from all organs, some have a more intimate connection to emotions; these are the heart and the liver. He furthermore outlined that because the heart influences the spirit and the sense of wellbeing, and the liver regulates the flow of blood and *qi*, these organs are dominant parts of human anatomy and their disturbance leads to serious illnesses.

Regarding the therapy of illnesses caused by emotions, all practitioners emphasized the importance of manual therapies like acupuncture. In accordance with the results of their anamnesis, they choose specific points for acupuncture or massage. However, the staff of Clinic A underlined that their clinic specifically applies relaxation training and conversational therapy. The vice-director Doctor Zhang explained that, beside acupuncture, he teaches patients exercises which they can do on their own in their daily life:

> For example, for people who are very nervous, I teach methods which will provide relaxation (*biru hen jinzhang de ren wo jiao yixie huanhe de fangfa* 比如很紧张的人我教一些缓和的方法). For people who are under pressure or depressed, I teach methods which will discharge pressure (*biru yali de ren, yumen de*

---

124 The history of this idiomatic expression (the Chinese term is chengyu 成语) goes back to the 12th century and roots in the poem man jiang hong 满江红 (trad. characters: 滿江紅) ("The River All Red"), presumably written by Yue Fei 岳飞 (1103-1142), who was a military general and poet. The expression nu fa chong guan 怒发冲冠 (trad. characters: 怒髮衝冠) is the first line of this poem, in which the author reflects the hatred he felt towards the combating Jin-Dynasty. Concerning Yue Fei and his later exploitation as a national hero, see Matten 2011.

ren wo jiao yixie xuanxie de fangfa 比如压力的人，郁闷的人我教一些宣泄的方法) (Interview with Dr. Zhang; Böke: Fieldwork 2010/2011).

These methods mainly consist of meditation and of creating a quiet and relaxed atmosphere, he outlined. A staff member of Clinic A explained in more detailed that, because emotions and the physical body are connected, they first analyse the reasons for the bodily symptoms (*zhe ge zhengzhuang shi cong na ge jihuan lai de* 这个症状是从那个疾患来的) and treat this bodily symptom accordingly (*shengli zhengzhuang zhiliao* 生理症状治疗). Afterwards, the patients are confronted with Chinese paintings, calligraphy or music which should serve as medium for meditation. This is said to create a calm and peaceful feeling (*pingjing anjing de ganjue* 平静安静的感觉). To support this, it is regarded as important for the practitioners to create an atmosphere of mutual trust (*xinren* 信任).

All practitioners stated that it is important to explain the disease and its causation to the patients in order to impart the knowledge of Chinese medical ideas concerning the preservation of health. However, as presented in a preceding paragraph, Chinese urban inhabitants do not recognize conversations with medical staff as an important source of medical knowledge.

In summary, one can say that the medical experts agree that theoretically all emotions can influence health, and all organs are possible victims of emotional disturbance. They additionally concur that the most dangerous emotion is anger, and the most vulnerable organs are the heart and the liver. These experts' estimations correspond with lay peoples' perceptions regarding emotions and illnesses.

Medical Experts' Estimations of Patients' Knowledge

I asked the medical experts, referring to their daily experience, to assess the knowledge of their patients regarding Chinese medical theory in general and regarding the connection between emotions and illness in particular. The experts all agree that there is a certain level of knowledge among the population of Beijing, both regarding general Chinese medical concepts and regarding the potential pathologic quality of emotions. However, there is a conflict in the appraisal of whether the knowledge was more extensive in former times or not. Whereas some doctors insists that in former times the knowledge of Chinese medicine among lay persons was better, others interject that due to the shrinking illiteracy rate in modern China, there is a better pervasion of knowledge among common people because they are now able to read books, newspapers and prescriptions.

Doctor Zhang emphasized the special role of Beijing in Chinese medicine, because for him, due to its several medical institutions, "Beijing is the best city for Chinese medicine in the whole country" (*beijing shi dui zhongguo zai quanguo zui hao de chengshi* 北京是对中医在全国最好的城市). However, he claimed that the knowledge of Chinese medical concepts and principles is not equally distributed among the common people. From his point of view, the common people recognise some general principles but "the doctor's knowledge is not spread widely enough" (*yishi renshi de hai bu guo shen* 医师认识的还不够申). Approximately half of his patients have reliable basic knowledge of Chinese medicine, but he claims that this is not representative of the whole urban population because normally, people acquaint themselves with Chinese medicine before visiting Chinese medical institutions. This view is supported by remarks stated by the staff of Clinic A, who also emphasized that patients normally familiarize themselves with Chinese medicine prior to consultation. They claimed that because Western medicine is the main trend (*xiyi shi zhuliu de* 西医是主流的), people without knowledge usually prefer Western medicine. However, this preference is not because of a truly free choice, but because of a lack of knowledge: when in doubt, people without experiences with Chinese medicine normally choose Western medicine because of its broader popularity.

Another medical expert, Doctor Wang, accentuated the speciality of Chinese medicine being a "folk medicine" (*minjian de yixue tixi*民间的医学体系). He explained that Chinese medicine is rooted in traditions (*chuantong xialai yixie dongxi* 传统下来一些东西) and characterized through trial and error (*changshi xing*尝试性). Therefore, Chinese medicine is a folk medicine (*zhongyi shi bijiao minjian de yixue tixi*中医是一种比较民间的医学体系), which can also be detected in the fact that there are many idiomatic expressions (*chengyu*成语) in Chinese which refer to ideas or observations rooted in Chinese medicine.[125] This is especially true for emotional states like 'anger' (*shengqi*生气) or 'hurriedness' (*zhaoji*着急). The pathological potential of these two emotions is perceived widely among common people, he explained.

Additionally, Doctor Li provided me with a closer look into patient's narration on illness episodes and on the declaration of symptoms. He explained that normally, his patients only complain about a vague indisposition (*bu shufu*

---

125 Also see for example Wierzbicka (1999), Pritzker (2003).

不舒服). Sometimes, patients furthermore emphasized insomnia (*shimian* 失眠), but they never complain about specific emotions or emotional distress.[126] However, he does not blame patients who actively hide their emotional distress, but claims that people do not know the influence of emotions on health (*ren bu liaojie qingxu de yingxiang* 人不了解情绪的影响).

Medical Experts' Position to Transfer of Knowledge

Regarding the transfer of knowledge, I was particularly interested in the perception of the expert's role in spreading medical knowledge and in their estimations of the famous TV infotainment shows which are, according to my survey results, the most important source of medical knowledge among common urban Chinese. To the first point, I already presented the perception stated by professionals that doctors are expected to explain the illness and its cause to the patient (see chapter 6). However, among the students of Chinese medicine I commonly received the answer that Chinese doctors regard themselves not as interpreters, but as specialists whose work is to cure the people from their ailments instead of explaining their craft. According to them, explaining the backgrounds is often considered to overstrain the patients. This view seems to coincide more with the common people's estimation of doctors as only a minor source of medical knowledge.

Asked to list the most important sources for common people to obtain medical knowledge, professionals listed, beside the conversation with doctors during consultation hour, print media, TV shows and internet resources (all also present in my survey results); however, they frequently stated additionally that especially young and well educated people join public lectures of doctors commonly given at university campuses (for example Doctor Zhang: "[they] take part in lectures and listen to doctors [explanations]" *canjia jiangzuo tingdao yisheng* 参加讲座听到医生 or Doctor Liang: "today the lectures on campuses have a big influence, at Beida[127], at Qinghua[128], they all have this [lectures]" *xianzai xuexiao jiaolou hen you yingxiang, beida, qinghua dou you* 现在学校教楼演讲很有影响，北大、清华都有). Moreover, Clinic A offers lectures for lay people in which professionals explain specific illnesses in detail,

---

126   c.f. chapter 5.
127   Beijing University (Beijing Daxue 北京大学), commonly refered to as Beida 北大.
128   Qinghua University (Qinghua Daxue 清华大学; in older transcription Tsinghua), commonly referred to as Qinghua 清华.

using medical textbooks as well as clinical studies and common people's everyday experiences. Beside the knowledge transfer, the focus of these lectures is especially oriented towards prevention of health and avoidance of illness.[129]

Concerning the TV infotainment shows, my informants were not unanimous on their actual benefit for patient's knowledge. On the one hand, all medical experts conceded that due to these shows, Chinese medicine gets more attention and the ideas and concepts of Chinese medicine are more present in common people's minds. Doctor Sun for example, stated that this kind of TV programme promotes Chinese medicine (*wo juede zhe zhong dianshi jiemu xuanchuan zhongyi* 我觉得这种电视节目宣传中医) and he added that these programmes are intelligible to the common people (*bijiao tongsu* 比较通俗). Even more positively answered Doctor Liu; from his point of view, only the best physicians appear on the TV screens and he judges their explanations as very good (*dianshishang de zhuanjia shi zui hao de, wo juede tamen shuo hen hao* 电视上的专家是最好的，我觉得他们说很好). However, other professionals were more reluctant in their evaluation of these TV shows. They emphasized the oversimplification of certain circumstances. For example, Doctor Zhou (Clinic B) criticised that in these shows there is a tendency to provide standard solution; this, she stressed, is completely against Chinese medical theory wherein every case is to be considered individually. Accordingly, the solutions presented on television are too simple and mislead people to think that cure is easily achievable. Other doctors faulted that in some of these shows the main interest is not in providing information on health and prevention, but doctors are eager to promote ready-made herbal drugs or have other monetary goals. One doctor told me that she heard a story that a physician in a TV show claimed to be able to cure cancer with specific infusions he prepares by himself. She remarked ironically that luckily for him, he sells these products in his own private clinic. So with the TV shows, he engages in advertisement both for his clinic and for his medical products.

---

129 I joined one of these lectures in spring 2011. The doctor lectured on common cold, provided insight in Chinese medical theories on the emergence of cold and gave instructions to prevention. The lecture was conducted in a special classroom located inside the clinic. The room was completely filled with participants, mainly women in their 40s or 50s. The whole lecture took one hour and I had the impression that it was not only a lecture on medical content but a kind of social event, gathering middle class urban inhabitants with a common interest, namely the preservation of health and wellbeing, and thereby improving and consolidate patient or 'customer' loyalty.

Concluding, one can say that in general Chinese medical experts appreciate the popularity which is created by TV shows and regard them as a tool to spread basic medical knowledge to common people. However, they additionally identify certain problems in these shows, ranging from oversimplification to moral conflicts. The accentuation of the doctor's important role in providing medical knowledge by contrast is opposed to common people's estimation.

Medical Experts' Statements on Group Specific Behaviour and Estimations

During my interviews with the medical professionals, certain age- or social-group specific topics regarding the clientele usually visiting Chinese medical institutions were omnipresent. Whereas only one doctor (Doctor Zhou, Clinic B) explained that there are no specific social groups or age cohorts visiting her consultation hours more often than others[130], all the other practitioners emphasized that during the last few years, they noticed an increase of younger people visiting the clinic with specific ailments. Their explanation for this process is two-part: the medical experts emphasized the younger generations' openness for Chinese medicine in contrast to older generations; furthermore, they also noticed ailments which are more present among younger urban inhabitants than among older people and which are considered to be curable by Chinese medicine.

Younger Generation's Openness for Chinese Medical Ideas

From Doctor Wang's point of view, older people "for historical reasons" (*zai zaoxian de shidai* 在早先的时代) trust more in Western medical concepts, because Western hospitals were the dominant form of medical institutions several years ago and they are more accustomed to it. On the other hand, among the younger generations he notices 'a resurgence' (*fuxing* 复兴) of Chinese medicine and these younger adults are more willing to engage the ideas of Chinese medicine (*geng rongyi jieshou zhongyi* 更容易接受中医). Doctor Sun also

---

130 Although towards the end of our interview she added that recently many "white-collar workers" (bailing 白领) came to their clinic suffering from work-related ailments like stress. However, she stressed that there are no special groups among her patients, old and young, richer and poorer, all are represented.

states that younger people are very interested in Chinese medicine (*nianqingren dui zhongyi hen gan xingqu* 年轻人对中医很感兴趣). He ascribes this interest to a more general interest in Chinese traditions, as he remarks laughingly that traditional or historical novels and TV soap operas are also very popular among younger people (*zai zhongguo nianqingren shou zhe zhong chuantong gudai xiaoshuo, dui zhe ge bijiao chuantong dianshiju hen gan xingqu* 在中国年轻人受这种传统古代小说，对这个比较传统的电视剧很感兴趣).

Referring to political and historical reasons, Doctor Liu explains that "in our history there was a thing called 'Cultural Revolution'" (*women de shang yi dai you yige shiqing jiao wenhua geming* 我们的上一代有一个事情交文化革命). During this period, he continued, cultural traditions were regarded as obsolete (*chuantong wenhua jiushi* 传统文化旧式); including Chinese medicine. People abandoned traditions and were educated according to Western science and technology (*zai nage shihou jiaoyu gen guanshu xifang keji* 在那个时候教育跟灌输西方科技), he explains; but for several years now, people have begun to realize that this Western science and technology is actually creating new problems for China and specific illnesses (*danshi jingguo duonianlai faxian xifang keji zai zhongguo zhi shenme wenti huo yizhun jibing* 但是经过多年来发现西方科技在中国致什么问题或一准疾病). Therefore, he concluded, younger people turn their attention back to traditional Chinese culture and on Chinese medicine (*suoyi nianqingren zhaodaole zhongguo chuantong wenhua he zhongyi* 所以年轻人找到了中国传统文化和中医).

A slightly different emphasis was expressed by Doctor Feng and Doctor Ding (Clinic C). They explained that younger urban inhabitants apply Chinese medicine not for curing illnesses in the first place, but mainly to abolish minor ailments which are closely connected to beauty or wellness, for example skin or hair problems or relaxation. These illnesses, they continued, are connected to emotions, because emotional distress often can cause problems like 'alopecia' (*tuofa* 脱发) or 'psoriasis' (*niupixian* 牛皮癣). Among their patients complaining about these and related illnesses, there is a dominant group they subsume under the label 'white-collar-worker' (*bailing* 白领). In this group, consisting mainly of younger to mid-aged middle class people, they identify a real 'hype' (*rechao* 热潮) for Chinese medicine as a cure for issues related to beauty and wellness.

Group Specific Ailments of Young Urban Inhabitants

All practitioners identified a set of circumstances which could be harmful for their clientele and which are connected to common perceptions of daily routine and lifestyle. They all agreed to the fact that modern lifestyle, especially in the big cities, creates an atmosphere of stress and pressure for younger people which are differentiated on several levels such as family or occupation.

Doctor Liu listed several kinds of pressure, which young people have to endure; the pressure of schooling and education, the pressure of occupation and the pressure of the family (*nianqingren yao kefu jiaoyu yali, zhiye yali, jiating yali* 年轻人要克服教育压力，职业压力，家庭压力). Especially regarding education, there is a huge pressure on students, he emphasized:[131]

> In Laozi's Daodejing there is a paragraph read like this: humans have five virtues, humanity, truthfulness, ritual [propriety], knowledge, and faithfulness, but for the development of society, humanity, truthfulness, ritual and faithfulness all have been lost. The last [item] remaining is knowledge.
>
> *Laozi zai daodejing you yi zhan shuo: 'ren you ren, yi, li, zhi, xin wu zhong pinde', danshi jiyu shenhui de fazhan ren, yi, li, xin dou shiqu le. Zhi sheng qilai zhi.*
> 老子在道德经有一章说：'人有仁、义、礼、知、信五种品德'，但是基于社会的发展仁、义、礼、信都失去了。只剩起来知。 (Interview with Dr. Liu; Böke: Fieldwork 2010/2011)

Consequently, knowledge is the way which has to be pursued for social advancement and thereby became a field of competition, creating stress and the other symptoms mentioned (see chapter seven for further discussion).

This view is supported by Doctor Sun's statements. He explained that the pressure is likely connected to the lifestyle (*keneng gen shenghuo fangshi you guanxi* 可能跟生活方式有关系) and that especially in the cities, there is a huge pressure created by conflicts around study or occupation (*zai da chengshi gongzuo, xuexi miandui hen da, suoyi tamen de yali hen da* 在大城市工作、学习面对很大，所以他们的压力很大). Older people already passed this period of life and, according to Doctor Sun, even if they are not yet retired, they often are well established in their jobs and settled with their families. He noticed an increase of illnesses related to pressure and stress during the

---

131 The attribution of this quotation to Laozi's Daodejing, a Daoist classic, is misleading. In fact, the listed virtues are Confucian virtues expressed in classics of the philosophical canon.

past few years and identifies the "rapid development" (*kuaisu fazhan* 快速发展) of society to be the reason for this increase. According to him, young people have to deal with 'contradictions' (*maodun* 矛盾) because there are many new ideas and ideals rapidly emerging (*you hen duo guannian, xinxian zhiyuan kuaisu de chuxian* 有很多观念、新鲜志愿快速额出现) which collide with older views.

Doctor Wang specified the generations in their 20s or 30s as being especially prone to suffer from these circumstances. He also listed work-related issues for stress and pressure; for example, they are very busy at work (*ren hen mang*人很忙), they have to work extra-hours (*jiaban* 加班) or have to go on business trips (*yao chuchai*姚出差). But he additionally blamed more socio-economic problems to be further triggers; namely he sees the problem of rising price level without equivalent increase in wages (*wujia hen zhang, danshi gongzi bu da*物价很涨，但是工资不大). Additionally, he criticised the insufficient pension scheme which forces younger generations to support the older, retired family members (*zhaobu laoren*找补老人), although they have children themselves which they have to care for (*gu ziji haizi* 顾自己孩子).

Others diagnosed a discrepancy between the wishes and plans for the future and the reality. Doctor Feng and Doctor Ding explained that in modern, urban China, younger people can now theoretically choose between different life plans because there is greater job diversity than in former times; but these plans, they criticise, often collide with reality. Hence, these people face competition on many levels of socio-economic life, which clashes with - their often - romantic fantasies of their desired future. Furthermore, they resumed, these individuals are normally raised as only-children due to the one-child-policy established in China in 1979. Therefore, they are used to being the centre of attention during childhood, which later creates problems with social interaction, where they have to compromise and prove capacity for teamwork which ultimately leads to pressure in social relations.

Doctor Song explained the two categories of illnesses in Chinese medicine, 'inner' and 'outer' causes (*neibu de yuanyin he waibu de yuanyin* 内部的原因，和外部的原因) and clarified that stress and sorrows belong to the first category (*yali shi neibu de, jiaolü ye shi neibu de*压力是内部的，焦虑也是内部的). He also criticises the fastness of modern lifestyle (*shenghuo gaosu de fazhan*生活高速得发展). In contrast to other experts, he added that Western medicine commonly has no solution for these kinds of problems (*xiyi meiyou banfa* 西医没有办法). Because many young people nowadays are interested in Chinese medicine (*xianzai hen duo nianqingren tebie gan xingqu* 现在很多年轻人特别感兴趣), they try Chinese medicine instead of other options to cure their ailments. This has increased the confidence in Chinese medicine notably compared to former times. (*xianzai dui zhongyi de xinren bi guoqu da da jigaole* 现在对中医的信任比过去大大极高了).

The velocity of societal change (*shehui de fanzhan su, tai kuai le* 社会的发展速,太快了) is, in Doctor Zhang's eyes, responsible for the increase of emotion-related diseases (*qingzhi jibing zengjia* 情志疾病增加) among younger people. He regretted that due to the rapid change of society, people sometimes get lost and cannot find the right direction anymore (*you de shihou renmen keneng zhaobudao zhe ge fangxiang* 有的时候人们可能找不到这个方向). This is especially true for younger people, he said, because they are more affected by these changes and feel more contradictions and thus pressure (*shenghuo maodun da, yali ye da* 生活矛盾大,压力也大).

The 'velocity of lifestyle' is a common topic in experts' explanations; Doctor Wen used this phrase to indicate the reasons for young people's ailments. She recalled that many of her patients complaint about this 'velocity of life', which ultimately results in pressure (*tamen juede shenghuo hen kuai, yali hen da* 他们觉得生活很快,压力很大). She speculated that China has become more and more similar to Western societies and states that Chinese society's health problems therefore also have become more and more similar to [psychological] problems in these societies. She compared it to the situation in Germany and called the problems of stress and depression not only a Chinese phenomenon, but an international one (*zhongguo qingkuang gen deguo chabuduo, yinwei zhezhong fazhan yuelaiyue guojihua, wenti shi yiyang de* 中国情况跟德国差不多,因为这种发展是越来越国际化,问题时一样的).

Miscellaneous

During the expert interviews, the practitioners stated several assertions which can not be subsumed in the already mentioned categories, but which I do not want to withhold. Mainly, these statements deal with the relationship of Chinese medicine and Western medicine. More concretely, these experts' statements focus on two topics: the interconnection of these medical systems in China and the growing popularity of Chinese medicine in Western societies like in Germany.

Regarding the relationship between Chinese and Western medicine in China, usually the practitioners stated that Western medicine is the mainstream medical system (*xiyi shi zhuliu* 西医是主流), at least in Beijing. They agreed on the benefits of Western medicine in emergency cases and intensive-care situation, demanding that everyone with severe injuries (for example after a car accident), broken bones or acute bleeding has to visit a Western clinic. With acute problems, the practitioners agreed that Chinese urban inhabitants commonly visit Western clinics, while chronic illnesses are usually thought of as being more curable with Chinese medicine.

The experts also indicated several structural differences between Chinese and Western medicine. For example, Doctor Zhang explained:

> [these medical systems] have a different cultural background, [they] have a different history, consequently, they are two different systems (*bu tong de wenhua beijing, bu tong de lishi, jiu shi liang zhong bu tong de tixi* 不同的文化背景，不同的历史，就是两种不同的体系). Western medicine focuses on illnesses; Chinese medicine means to heal the [whole] human being; Chinese medicine means to teach balance (*xifang yixue jibing weizhu, zhongyi shi zhi ren, zhongyi shi tiaohe zhidao* 西方医学疾病为主，中医是治人，中医是调和指导). Western medicine does not balance human's lifestyle (*xiyi bu tiaohe renmen shenghuo xingwei* 西医不调和人们生活行为) (Interview with Dr. Zhang; Böke: Fieldwork 2010/2011).

Doctor Wen pointed in the same direction when she explained that Chinese medicine is looking for the root of the illness (*zhongyi renwei ben*中医认为本), whereas Western medicine only focuses on the illness itself (*xiyi jiaodian jiu shi bing* 西医焦点就是病). For Doctor Li, Chinese and Western medicine are also two inherently different perspectives (*xiyi he zhongyi shi liang bu tong de jiaodu* 西医和中医是两不同的角度), which he outlines in four points: first, Chinese medicine is focused on the 'immaterial' or the 'invisible' (*wuxing de dongxi* 无形的东西), in contrast to Western medicine; second, Chinese medicine views the human being as a unity (*zhongyi kan ren shi yi ge zhengpi* 中医看人是一个整批); third, he described Chinese medicine as focusing on the adjustment of the body (*zhongyi shi tiaoli tiaoji* 中医是调理调剂), while Western medicine mainly proposes intervention (*ganyu* 干预); and finally, Doctor Li identifies the emphasis of prevention (*yufang* 预防) in Chinese medicine, while Western medicine (according to him) has to wait until the illness occurs. Another common statement was the characterization of Chinese medicine as free of side-effects (*meiyou fuzuoyong* 没有副作用).

All practitioners traced the growing popularity of Chinese medicine in Western societies with sympathy. Dr. Liang for example stated that, although there are differences, both systems could learn from each other, because, as she continues "both systems are good and they have a common goal, namely the overcoming of illnesses" (*zhongyi ye hao, xiyi ye hao, mudi jiu shi jibing jiejue* 中医也好，西医也好，目的就是疾病解决). Because of Chinese medicine's emphasis on the root of the illness, its low rates of side effects and its advantages in treating chronicle diseases, she appreciates the spread of Chinese medicine in Western societies. The medical staff of Clinic A pointed to the fact that Chinese medicine has already been successfully exported to Japan and Korea and therefore expected no difficulties in the transformation into Western societies. The experts agreed that Chinese medicine, for the benefit of all humans, should be transported into other societies. Doctor Zhang emotively stated that "Chinese medicine does not belong to just one people or nation, but belongs to humankind" (*zhongyi bu shuyu minzu huozhe guojia, danshi shuyu renlei* 中医不属于民族或者国家，但是属于人类).

However, practitioners not only emphasized the advantages of spreading Chinese medicine in Western societies, but also stated that they benefited from several achievements of Western medicine. Doctor Sun explained that in general, diagnostics are valued as good and beneficial, while technology and devices used commonly in Western medicine are also practically applicable to Chinese medicine. He praised imaging procedures such as x-ray as important and helpful to Chinese medicine and explained that for example, electrocardiogram could facilitate and complement traditional Chinese pulse diagnostic.

7. Specific Answering Patterns

In this chapter I combine the results of the survey with the expert interviews and analyse three main realms which emerged during the empirical phase of my work: first, age-specific peculiarities; second, education-specific peculiarities; and third, gender-specific peculiarities. It is worthwhile to analyse these three major domains in detail because the survey results and thus the common peoples' estimations as well as the experts' views all point in the same direction. In the subsequent paragraphs, these three domains are elaborated upon, complemented with explanatory approaches and linked to philosophical and sociological discourses on power and capital.

Age-specific Peculiarities: Changing Habitus and Different Modes of Power

Throughout the whole study, one can detect that age is an important variable for the estimation of certain aspects of Chinese medicine: younger Chinese urban inhabitants faced the questionnaire more openly and were more confident regarding their knowledge of Chinese medicine compared to older people.[132] This is not an emic impression; medical practitioners also regarded younger Chinese to be more interested in traditional elements of Chinese culture and therefore also more open to Chinese medicine than older people.

Asking about illnesses caused by emotions, older people listed different illnesses than younger people, focusing more on 'somatic' ailments like heart disease while neglecting 'psychological' issues. Medical experts reported that during consultation, older people usually present 'somatic' complaints instead of 'psychological' problems.

During interviews, the informants routinely referred to "specific historic conditions", "totally different historical background" or to "a certain period in history", emphasizing that experience of history has relevance for today's estimations and attitudes. Chinese people have faced radical changes of society and the political system in the 20th century. During the first half of the century, a deep transformation of Chinese society proceeded, starting with the abolition of

---

132 This is not significant in the analysis on my quantitative data, but the qualitative interviews with lay people and also with medical experts all hint on it.

the Chinese Empire and the foundation of the republic, the occupation by the Japanese Empire, the civil war and the implementation of the People's Republic in 1949. Although on the surface the political system stayed the same during the second half of the last century, again society had to endure deep changes initiated through political campaigns like the 'Great Leap Forward' (1958-1961), the 'Cultural Revolution' (1966-1976) and the 'Open Door Policy (1978). At least since Pierre Bourdieu's "Habitus" (1979) and Thomas Csordas' "Embodiment" (1990) it is common sense in Cultural Anthropology that historic experiences manifest themselves not only in the way people act or talk, but also directly in the body.[133] Crossley (2001: 93) explains, making recourse to Bourdieu, that

> an agent's habitus is an active residue or sediment of their past experience which functions within their present, shaping their perception, thought and action and thereby shaping social practice.

Aesthetic as well as ethic or normative dispositions of one's social space are internalized at an early age and work throughout a lifetime. The body and its functions are not only an object in relation to culture, but a subject of culture. Some other anthropological studies in the context of Chinese medicine, especially those by Susan Greenhalgh (for example 1994, 2001, 2008), already worked out the specific influence of the political environment in China on the body and on further medical issues. I try to adhere to this view and exemplify some of the theories which assume a link between political and societal power and the medical sector based on the findings of my study.

The Suspiciousness of Older Generations and the "Hype" of Chinese Medicine Among Younger Urban Inhabitants

Throughout the whole survey, I found behavioural patterns which I like to call age-specific: older people in their 50s or older, although helpful and pleased about my interest in Chinese medicine, answered spontaneously that they do not know much about this topic. These people reflexively pointed to other people around which, in their eyes, had better knowledge of Chinese medicine and advised me to ask these people. This behaviour was almost never seen among

---

[133] Although one can interpose that Cultural Anthropology already knew Marcel Mauss' "Technique du corps" (1935) and Mary Douglas' "Two Bodies" (1973), Bourdieu and Csordas seized on their ideas and elaborated these theories.

younger generations. The latter, in contrast, confidently answered my questions and conveyed a feeling of interest in Chinese medicine. There are two possibilities of explaining this age-specific behaviour: first, the scepticism of older generation on the one hand and the openness and self-confidence of the youth on the other could be interpreted in the broader context of a younger generation more familiar and curious about foreigners, more acquainted to international phenomena and therefore more open in interviews with foreign researchers. The second explanation emphasises the younger generation's interest in 'Chinese traditional culture'. Although, as already outlined in the preceding chapter, the analysis of quantitative data reveals no significant evidence that younger generations know Chinese medical concepts like the 'Six Evils' or the 'Seven Emotions' better than older people; however, the qualitative interviews with medical experts support my impression that the young people in their 20s and 30s are the main devotees of Chinese medicine in contemporary urban China. With the exception of one doctor, all the others emphasized firmly the youth's interest in everything connected to an impression of 'Chinese traditional culture' and hence the growing relevance of Chinese medicine in these cohorts, while they frequently labelled older generations as more sceptical and reluctant towards everything 'old' and 'traditional'. The explanation is connected to specific personal and collective historical experiences.[134]

Older generations experienced the already mentioned "specific historical conditions". We do not have to speculate about the excessive events and persecution during Cultural Revolution. In these prevailing times, the everyday experience of abolition of traditional culture, manifested in the destruction of architecture, in the burning of books or in the equation of tradition and feudalism offers sufficient evidence to comprehend the older people's reluctance to TCM; "Delegitimation spread from a crisis of confidence in the political system to a wholesale questioning of the major indigenous cultural institutions" (Kleinman & Kleinman 1994: 713). Zhang and Schwartz open a window in the time of the Cultural Revolution, by quoting their informant's memories: "there was a campaign against the Four Olds: old thought, old culture, old tradition, and old custom" (Zhang & Schwartz 2003: 111).[135] Hence, it is understandable that older people still feel uncomfortable with topics related to these former 'Four Olds'.

---

134 I refer to Connerton 1989 for a decisive description of 'remembering societies', were he exemplifies that societies remember in three different ways: first, through inscription (in myths, books, monuments etc.), second, by commemorative rituals, and third, via incorporation of social memory into the human body (c.f. Kleinman & Kleinman 1994: 707).

135 The campaign to "destroy the four olds" (po si jiu 破四旧) was one of the first campaigns during Cultural Revolution. For this early phase of the Cultural Revolution, see Wang 2003.

This view was also expressed by the medical experts. They all, with the exception of one, referred to this period in Chinese history, either directly by naming it or indirectly by describing it as "specific historic experience". Several discussions with Chinese university graduates supported this interpretation.

Obviously, younger Chinese do not share this experience of abandoning important indigenous cultural institutions. People in their 20s or 30s are raised under the political slogan "getting rich is glorious" (*zhifu guangrong* 致富光荣)[136] initiated in the late 1970s and experienced the Open Door Policy of Deng Xiaoping and his successors. For this generation, class struggle is not on the political agenda anymore. Instead, the recent Chinese leaders guided China in a new, capitalist way which lead to rising economic and living standards, bringing along totally different conditions and, beside other difficulties, new medical problems. The pragmatic handling of the ideology of Deng and his followers is best presented in Deng's widely quoted statement that "it doesn't matter if the cat is black or white, as long as it catches mice, it is a good cat" (*buguan hei mao bai mao zhuadao laoshu jiu shi hao mao* 不管黑猫白猫抓到老鼠就是好猫).[137] Growing nationalism and the rediscovery of 'traditional Chinese culture' is not only allowed, but encouraged by the political elite. In this climate, as Doctor Sun in an expert interview remarked, 'traditional' coated things such as TV soap operas superficially playing in the old imperial China, or Chinese medicine, which in its official English translation is called "Traditional Chinese Medicine" (see Chapter 1), are very popular among young urban Chinese. Younger patients are described as more interested in and more open to Chinese medical theory and therapy by all practitioners I interviewed. During many conversations with informants they stated that younger Chinese are interested in the cultural heritage of their predecessors and Chinese medicine is widely conceived as being part of Chinese cultural legacy which one has to admire with pride and loyalty.[138]

Antagonistic Estimation of Stress and Depression

According to the presented empirical data, depression and stress at first sight seem to be problems only affecting the younger generations. People in their 60s

---

136 Quoted from Rojek 2001: 89.
137 Quoted from Rojek 2001: 96.
138 For a description of the specific kind of "Filial nationalism" among Chinese urban youth see Fong 2004.

or older do not regard stress or pressure as potentially pathogenic emotions and do not perceive depression as an illness category in the field of emotion-related illnesses. However, as already pointed out, different studies revealed that depression, at least diagnosed according to a biomedical paradigm, is prevalent among Chinese older people, too (for example Phillips et al 2009, Chen et al. 2005, Sun 2004).

Obviously there are some stressors which are almost exclusively influencing younger people. These are, as also identified by medical experts, stressors regarding the foundation and maintenance of a family as well as starting and maintaining a professional career. These stressors work for women as well as for men, although to a different extent. (I summarize the gender-dimension of these stressors at the end of this subchapter). The perception of work and family foundation as stressors in Chinese society is not a totally new phenomenon, as Lin & Lai in the early 1990s already identified both as present challenges and demands to the individual (Lin & Lai 1995). But in addition to their findings, I would like to argue that in the 2010s, the pressure has increased. The state-run enterprises, which at least conveyed a weak idea of security and social support, are being liquidated, and with the liquidation of these working units (*danwei* 单位), also the 'iron-rice-bowl', which "symbolized the Communist party's commitment to provide cradle-to-the-grave security for all its citizens" (Hughes 2002: ix), disappeared.

Consequently, a new, more open but less secure economic landscape emerged in China. Additionally, the 'traditional' norm for adults to get married and to begin a family, which Lai (1995: 12) noticed for the 1990s, is still an imperative. And again, things have changed during the last 20 years and increased the pressure and stress. In former times, only boys received an adequate education, because they were thought of being the future head of the family. Due to the One-Child-Policy, men and women are now both competing with each other for higher education and prestigious jobs as education of daughters is no longer regarded as waste of money and dedication (c.f. Fong 2002). Additionally, boys were considered to be the supporters of the parents when they retired, an imperative of a concept which is called 'filial piety' (*xiao* 孝)[139]. Previously, the conducting of specific rituals related to this concept and the caring for the older family member was a duty of the sons. In modern China, due to the One-Child-Policy this has to be implemented now both by the one son or the one daughter. On the one hand this can be valuated as a sign of gender equality, on the other hand it obviously conflicts with young people's wishes to an independent and

---

[139] An overview about the concept of filial piety in East Asia and especially in China offers the collection of essays by Ikels (2004).

self-determined life, not to mention the possible economic difficulties of sustaining the in-laws (c.f. Fong 2007:93-95).

In former times, girls, as they married into a 'new' family, were not regarded as being able to lead a family and support the parents. Yan (2006: 106) portrays the role of the young women drastically:

> Young women were marginal outsiders with only a temporary position, as daughters married out and new daughters-in-law entered the domestic group [...]. Thus, daughters were commonly regarded as a drain on family wealth and new daughters-in-law were seen as a potential thread to the existing family order. In comparison to their male siblings, girls were statusless, powerless, and somewhat dangerous.

However, Fong (2002) describes excellently how opinions regarding daughters' ability to guarantee 'piety' changed during the last decades, because the One-Child-Policy eliminated the competition between brothers and sisters for education and restricted the choice of parental support and investment which ultimately benefited the girls.[140] For the same reason, women are now freer in mate selection than they have been in Chinese history. In the urban area, arranged marriage nowadays is totally uncommon (Whyte 1997: 3)[141] and women are the primary agent of partner choice.[142] Chinese women are eager to marry 'upward'

---

140 Jankowiak et al (2012) explain that especially in rural China daughters are regarded as being „more economically beneficial" (80) due to the increased bride prices. Additionally, they are characterized as „being more loyal and emotionally involved with their natal familiy" (ibid). However, I doubt the conclusion of the authors that „daughters are tacitly replacing sons as the preferred gender" (ibd.). Instead of tacit replacement, I would rather call it a 'tacit equalization'.

141 This is a rather new development. Lang (1946: 122-124) shows that in the 1930s, the majority of students as well as industrial workers in an Chinese urban setting were not involved in mate selection and not seldom even had not seen their future spouse before the wedding. For the 1960s, Whyte & Parish (1984: 119) explain that although free mate selection already had won general acceptance among the urban population, almost 50% of the couples in their sample did not meet directly, but had to rely on introductions, either by parents or by friends or workmates.

142 Xia & Zhou (2003: 237-238) write: "wealth, advanced academic degrees, and body height are most important for Chinese women today [...]. Women have higher expectations for men's emotional commitment. They want quality marriages with high emotional compatibility, sexual enjoyment, and freedom to act independently. They want husbands with great self-cultivation, social status, reputation and wealth [...]". For a special form of female agency in marriage, the bargaining and control of bridewealth. see Yan 2005.

on the social ladder; this doubtlessly creates pressure for both sexes because women are now forced to meet a certain ideal as well as represent specific social and bodily features in order to impress socially higher mates. They have to be "beautiful, healthy, gentle, chaste, and youthful" (Xia & Zhou 2003: 237). It also creates pressure for men, as they are under the more principal pressure of finding a future bride among their social peers. As women seek to marry 'upward', 'lower class' men are running out of potential mates, an effect which is even increased by the specific Chinese birth-rate: the number of boys born per 100 girls measures 120, creating far-reaching social problems (Greenhalgh 2011: 160; for the problem of infanticide and the "missing girls of China" also see Ebenstein 2010). Both sexes have in common that not only must they support their own child in every possible way to foster a 'superior child' (see chapter 7), the additionally have to support the parents of both spouses; a moral obligation according to the concept of piety, but also a vital necessity because of the insufficient Chinese pension scheme. As a result of the One-Child-Policy, often there are no siblings to share this burden; an issue which was also stated in an expert interview with Doctor Wang. A study by Zhan (2006) reveals that care giving children of aging parents more often suffer from stress and depression than others.

These problems of finding a suitable mate and supporting both children and parents dramatically collide with emerging new family ideas of pursuing intimacy, independence, free choice and individual happiness (Yan 2009: XXIV; for the situation in the countryside, see Yan 2003) which consequently leading to stress and pressure.

Beside these rather age-specific conditions, it can be assumed that further predicaments like a change in lifestyle and a general acceleration of life, especially perceptible in an urban environment, must be experienced by all age groups; this was also the conclusion drawn by most of the medical experts I interviewed. So there is still a lack of explanation as to why older people did not perceive stress and depression to be relevant factors in emotional instability. This leads us again the question of 'somatization' (also see chapter 5).

'Somatization' versus 'Psychologization'

As already pointed out earlier, 'somatization' was thought of being the "chief idiom through which Chinese culture articulates [...] neurotic disorders" (Lin et al. 1980: 253). For my study I not only recognized the tendency to 'somatize' among older survey participants, but also during my interviews with medical experts this topic was on the agenda. Doctors also explained that older people usually prefer the description of somatic symptoms rather than mentioning psychological distress, and request somatic therapy instead of psychological help. Accordingly, the medical experts stated that there are obviously pragmatic reasons for the older people's preference of somatic complaints: they explained that these complaints are simply more relevant for this age group, as they suffer more from somatic ailments like high blood pressure or heart disease than the younger generations.[143] However, I did not ask about concrete, personal illnesses, but about general connections between emotions and organs as well as about illnesses caused by emotions in general. Doctor Feng and Doctor Ding explained during interviews that old people and young people talk in their specific language, using specific vocabulary and express the symptoms according to their own cognitive schema: older people use 'somatic' expressions, physical symptoms to describe their ailments, whereas younger patients commonly refer to 'psychological' states or to emotional disturbance. Consequently, there is no 'right' or 'wrong', they pointed out. Older people are influenced by their historic experience, thus bringing together depression with insanity and regarding depression as very dangerous, because of a cultural stigma which equates depression with insanity, and because of a historic experience, where depression additionally carried a political stigma.

It is worthwhile to explain the older people's specific connotation of depression as dangerous, learned out of lessons which my informants frequently labelled as "specific historical experiences", with recourse to theoretical considerations about 'power', 'ruling' and 'governing', because, as Rose (2011: 250) puts it, "China's move towards a market economy in the 1980s was coupled with changes in the organisation of political power". By considering this sphere with Michel Foucault, I try to apply parts of his theoretical framework to underpin the body of my empirical data and hope to open a window for further research on the connection and interaction of illness concepts, stigmas, power and "governmentality".

---

143 However, there are numerous hints for an increase of diseases of affluence among Chinese children and adolescents, resulting in obesity, diabetes, high blood pressure and so on (for example see Ji & Cheng 2008 or Lin et al. 2007).

Different modes of power

Governmentality, as Zhang (2011a: 1) remarks, was "raised by Foucault three decades ago at the same time as China's reform was about to start". He continues explaining that "governmentality is both a mode of power and a rationale for the use of power under modernity" and postulates that "the change in the relationship people have with the state in China has a lot to do with the deepening of governmentality, seen in the changing governance of life" (ibid. 1-2).

Foucault (1994a: 655) defined "governmentality" his lecture "Sécurité, territoire et population" at the Collège de France, Paris, in 1978 as follows:[144]

"Par gouvernementalité, j'entends l'ensemble constitué par les institutions, les procedures, analyses er réflexions, les calculs et les tactiques qui permettent d'exercer cette forme bien spécifique, bien que complexe, de pouvoir, qui a pour cible principale la population, pour forme majeure de savoir, l'économie politique, pour instrument technique essentiel les dispositifs de sécurité. Deuxièment, par <<gouvernementalité>>, je entends la tendance, la ligne de force qui, dans tour l'Occident, n'a pas cessé de conduire, et depuis fort longtemps, vers la prééminence de ce type de pouvoir qu'on peut appeler le <<gouvernement>> sur tous les autres: souverainité, discipline; ce qui a amené, d'une part, le développement de toute une série d'appareils specifiques de gouvernement et, d'autre part, le développement de toute une série de savoirs. Enfin, par gouvernementalité, je crois qu'il faudrait entendre le processus ou, plutôt, le résultat de processus par lequel l'Etat de justice de Moyen Âge, devenu aux XVe et XVIe siècles État administratif, s'est trouvé petit à petit <<gouvernementalisé>>.[145]

---

144 In French, almost all of Foucault's shorter writings, published interviews and miscellany have been published in a collection called Dits et écrits, originally published in four volumes in 1994, and which I quote here. In English, there are a number of overlapping anthologies, which often use conflicting translations of the overlapping pieces, frequently with different titles. Consequently, throughout this whole chapter I present the French original quote and a working translation of the paragraphs translated by myself.

145 "I understand governmentality as a sum total of institutions, procedures, analysises and reflections, the calculations and tactics, which allow the exercise of this specific, yet complex form of power. Its main aim is the population, its main form of knowledge is political economie, and its main technical instruments are the dispositifs de sécurité (apparatuses of security). Additionally, I understand governmentality as the tendency or line of force, which in the whole occident continually and since a very long time led to the primacy of a mode of power which may be termed ' to govern', in contrast to all other modes of power such as sovereignity and discipline. This resulted on the one hand in the development of a specific governance apparatus, on the other hand created new forms of savoir (knowledge). Finally I think that governmentality is to be seen as a pro-

He identified two antagonistic modes of power: first, ruling or sovereignty; and second, governing or governmentality. Whereas kings, monarchs, or dictators act as sovereigns and conduct the power of ruling, a modern state acts as government and conducts the power of governing. Kings or dictators rule by insuring the safety of their territory, consolidating their sovereignty and controlling territory and people (Foucault 2003: 802-810). Through the emergence of a "politic of force", power works on the individual body, on its parts, its gestures and its behaviour, calculating and manipulating (Foucault 2011:162); in contrast, to govern means to "improve the condition of the population, to increase its wealth, its longevity, and its health" (Foucault 2007: 105, in Zhang 2011: 11). It is my effort to show that not only in early modern Western states, as Foucault described it, a transformation of power from a purely 'ruling' sovereignty to a merely 'governing' governmentality happened. Also in China there was a shift in the execution of power after the death of Mao Zedong and the emergence of the Open Door Policy in the late 1970s, namely to mitigate the sovereignty of the Central State and to intensify the governmentality, which is reflected in my empirical data.

In the history of the People's Republic, certain political campaigns like the Great Leap Forward and the Cultural Revolution unveiled a specific insight into power relationships. Zhang explains that decision making during these periods was totally dominated by "revolutionary will and ideological passion" (Zhang 2011a: 7). There was "considerable pressure exerted, indirectly via state propaganda or directly via party cadres" (Powell & Cook 2000: 83) to ensure that people meet the official party ideal. Direct commands by representatives of the ideological leadership and "mass campaigns as elements of sovereignty" (Greenhalgh 2011: 157) were the primary enforcement of power. "Elements of governmental reason were engulfed by Maoist sovereignty and revolutionary frenzy" (Zhang 2011a: 3). Sanctions for misbehaviour were mostly public, so called 'class enemies' were pilloried and subjected to physical abuse in public (Fig. 33).

---

cess or the result of a process, through which the state of justice of the Middle Ages, transformed into the administrative state during the fifteenth and sixteenth centuries, step by step becomes 'governmentalized'" (my translation).

159

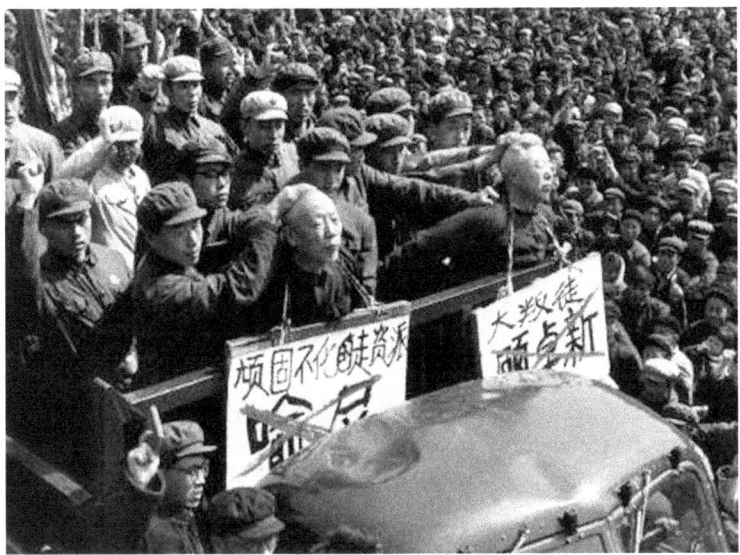

Fig. 33: Picture of a so called 'struggle session' taken in 1967 in Shenyang. On the placard around the necks of the two captives, the accusations are written: "narrow-minded capitalist ('capitalist roader') unwilling to change" (wangu bu hua de zouzipai 顽固不化的走资派) on the left placard; "gross traitor" (da pantu 大叛徒) on the right placard. The names of the men, written below the accusations, are crossed out, a typical sanction during Cultural Revolution (c.f. Lu 2004: 14).[146]

This kind of sanction comes close to what Foucault recognized as one marker of pre-modern ruling or sovereignty, illustrated in his introduction to his "naissance de la prison" (2011 [1975]), where he uses the description of the cruel torture and execution of delinquents performed in public to explain that the committed crime is not only an assault on the concrete victim, but always also an assault on the sovereign. It is a personal assault on the sovereign, as it attacks his will, and it is a physical assault, as the power of the law and the (physical) power of the sovereign is one. Therefore, the cruel punishment is a direct counterattack on the offender; or as Foucault phrases it, "une réplique directe à celui qui l'a offensé" (Foucault 2011: 59). Additionally, the offender, in pre-modern Europe as well as in revolutionary China, had to carry the indictment written on a board around his

---

146 Photography taken from boxun.com, an overseas Chinese community website widely considered to be an alternative source of news from China. http://news.boxun.com/news/gb/z_special/2009/08/200908120714.shtml, last access 08.06.2012.

neck, because "mais il s'agit aussi de rappeler que dans tout crime il y a comme un soulèvement contre la loi et que le criminel est un ennemi de prince" (ibid. 61).[147] However, it is not merely revenge, but has a political function, i.e. to restore the infringed sovereignty of the ruler by not recreating a balance, but by restoring the asymmetry between the subject who dared to infringe upon the law and the almighty ruler inherent in this system (Foucault 2011: 58-59).

Against this background, it is understandable that the notion of depression among older people is very specific; they witnessed times in which depression was thought of as rooting in false political attitude, for a true and confident socialist could *per definitionem* not be depressed, and therefore experiencing depression was equated with being a criminal directly attacking the sovereign, Mao Zedong or the Communist Party. One may intervene here and state that in modern China indeed there is, although limited through financial means and local access, a free choice of medical institutions and therapy. But, as Lukes (2005: 25-26) puts it

> Decisions are choices consciously and intentionally made by individuals between alternatives, whereas the bias of the system can be mobilized recreated and reinforced in ways that are neither consciously chosen nor the intended result of particular individuals' choices. [...] Moreover, the bias of the system is not sustained simply by a series of individually chosen acts, but also, most importantly, by the socially structured and culturally patterned behaviour of groups [...].

Additionally, to bring in Bourdieu's theory of habitus, different conditions of existence produce different forms of habitus, which in return means that

> An agent's whole set of practices (or those of a whole set of agents produced by similar conditions) are both systematic, inasmuch as they are the product of the application of identical (or interchangeable) schemes, and systematically distinct from the practices constituting another life-style (Bourdieu 2010: 166).

Lash (1991: 258) summarizes when he writes on Foucault's and Nietzsche's conception of memory that "punishment and discipline, through a sort of socialization process, create a 'memory' for offenders and for society in general".

---

147 "it must be remembered that every crime is also an upheaval against the law and that the criminal is an enemy of the prince [ruler]" (my translation).

That is exactly what the persecution of depression as a marker of counterrevolutionary attitude created.

However, in my opinion, not only the older generations' attitude on depression is rooted in the specific modes of power these generations have experienced, but also modern attitudes on depression are deeply connected with modern modes of power.

Foucault (2005: 48) stated in 1980 that in China, individual life is under most intensive control and that the state is interested in every aspect of the individual's life, and Susan Greenhalgh elucidated that with the death of Mao Zedong in 1976 "the governmentalization of population has proceeded rapidly" (Greenhalgh 2011: 158).[148] The new programmatic orientation of the Chinese government towards economic growth and increasing living standard needed this new mode of power, because, according to Foucault, the old power of 'ruling' characterizing dictatorship had negatively influences on economic processes:

> Le pouvoir était alors essentiellement percepteur et prédateur. Dans cette mesure, il opérait toujours une soustraction économique et, par conséquent, loin de favoriser et de stimuler le flux économique, il était perpétuellement son obstacle et son frein. D'où cette seconde preoccupation, cette seconde nécessité: trouver un mécanisme de pouvoir tel que, en meme temps qu'il contrôle les choses et les personnes jusqu'au moindre detail, il ne soit pas onéreux ni essentiellement prédateur pour la société, qu'il s'exerce dans le sens du processus èconomique lui-même.[149] (Foucault 1994b: 190).

The first and most prominent field of "biopolitical governance" (Greenhalgh 2011: 146) Chinese society had to face was the implementation and control of the One-Child-Policy.[150] Although not a direct matter of concern for my study, the consequences of this policy created a type of Chinese urban citizen which Greenhalgh calls "the neoliberal subject par excellence" (ibid. 155) and a "self-governing subject" (ibid. 156). This self-governing subject conceives a mission

---

148 This is not to say that aspects of governmentality in China were totally absent during Mao's lifetime. Examples are illustrated in Yang 2011 and partly in Zhang 2011b.
149 "Power took something away and was merely marauding. It always caused economic decrease. It did not encourage and stimulate economy, but interfered and restricted. Therefore another reason to find a mode of power which controls humans and things into every detail, but does neither incriminate nor despoil society, but works in the same direction as the economic process" (my translation).
150 Again I refer to the numerous works by Susan Greenhalgh cited above.

and a duty to maximise one's quality and to improve health to the best possible condition (Rose 2011: 251). By doing so, the subject not only makes the most of its individual capacities, but also supports the improvement of the health and quality of the whole Chinese people. This duty to be well is an important aspect of what Rose, in succession of Foucault, calls "biological citizenship" (Rose ibid. 237, also see Rose 2007, Rose & Novas 2005). He continues that this new doctrine of individuals' responsibility for health and wellbeing integrated on the one hand language and criteria of Euro-American ethical - and one may add here, biomedical - doctrine, and on the other hand also made recourse to indigenous traditions such as Confucianism or Daoism (ibid. 251). Evidently, this is true for my informants being in their 20s or 30s; they complain of stress and depression as the drawbacks of modern, cosmopolitan, urban lifestyle and thus seeking relaxation and healing in Chinese medicine. These cohorts of informants, as well as Rose's prototypical 'biological citizens',

> are managing their own biological capacities, [...] utilising multiple explanatory models to understand their health status, and multiple medical technologies, from herbal remedies and acupuncture through to traditional forms of bodily exercise and corporeal training to manage their own vital existence (ibid. 253).

Depression is no longer a condition which is sanctioned by a sovereign or dictator, but a problem rooting in the new, urban lifestyle, a lifestyle that according to Rose is best described as "regulated freedom" (ibid. 255). This problem of depression, according to my younger informants' views as well as according to medical experts' valuations, has to be, and can be, solved in institutions which Foucault identified as implementing the new power of governing more subtly than the ruler's public campaigns and public cruelties. These institutions, among others, are hospitals, clinics and doctors' offices (c.f. Foucault 2011: 200-227), through which the governing state demonstrates its existence by fostering and extending life (Zhang 2011: 11). However, this is not totally altruistic, because it is also part of the governmental power not merely to rule its subjects, but instead to govern a population; and this population is not just a group of people, but a group of humans, biological organisms regulated through certain processes and regularities (Foucault 1994b: 193).

> On s'aperçoit, par conséquent, que la relation de pouvoir avec le sujet ou, mieux, avec l'individu, ne doit pas être simplement cette forme de sujétion qui permet au pouvoir de prélever sur le sujet des biens, des richesses et éventuellement son corps

et son sang, mais que le pouvoir doit s'exercer sur les individus en tant qu'ils constituent une espèce d'entité biologique qui doit être prise en consideration, si nous voulons précisément utiliser cette population comme machine pour produire, pour produire des richesses, des biens, produire d'autres individus.[151]

The older generations, under the impression of sovereignty and dictatorship, have embodied the idea that depression is not an ailment in the first place, but a political offense committed against the ruler or sovereign. Therefore they habitually avoid considering it. Younger generations however, impressed by a different mode of power, are 'governed' through medical institutions in order to decrease their stress and depression for the sake of the individual as well as for the sake and development of the whole society. Or to speak with Alain Ehrenberg (2010 [1998]: 4)[152]:

> Depression began its ascent when the disciplinary model for behaviours, the rules of authority and observance of taboos that gave social classes as well as both sexes a specific destiny, broke against norms that invited us to undertake personal initiative by enjoying us to be ourselves.

Education-specific Peculiarities: Stress, Depression and the Chinese Education System

Stress, pressure and depression were commonly regarded as a problem by my informants, especially for young, well-educated urban dwellers. This hypothesis not only results from the analysis of quantitative data, which alone would not lead to robust results, but in considering the qualitative data as well, one gets enough indications for the connection between good education and prevalence for stress, pressure and depression. In informal interviews conducted during the

---

151 "The connection between the power and the subject, or better the individual, should not be limited to submission, allowing the power to take goods, wealth, and maybe even blood or live of the subject, but should focus on the individual as a biological, which has to be considered in order to use the population as production apparatus for generating wealth, goods and more individuals" (my translation).

152 Although his book "La Fatigue d'être soi" (1998) mainly analyzes the upcoming of depression in an Europeen context, it reveals significant parallels to the situation in contemporary China.

survey as well as during the interviews with medical experts informants frequently stated that "good education means high pressure" (*xueli gao, yali da* 学历高，压力大) and identified this with a specific group of urban inhabitants, namely university students or young university graduates.[153]

In a 1998 published article, Reed asked whether the ascetic and frugal socialist role model Lei Feng (雷锋)[154] is "dead for Chinese students", a common phrase she recorded on the streets of Beijing in the mid 1980s (Reed 1998: 359). She analysed that due to rising consumerism and rapid social, political and economic change, this old role model did not serve well anymore and had to be reshaped or replaced by something else, representing "the diversity and maturity of present-day Chinese youth and the fact that they 'have their own ideas'" (ibid. 364). Consequently, education changed from a collective brought-into-line learning into an individual-centred competition for best starting positions.

Maurer-Fazio (2006: 215) analysed that in the late 1990s, good education had become a key factor for successful labour market outcome, not only in sectors with high educational standards, but also for workers. My informants, both the common people I talked to on the streets as well as the medical experts I interviewed, all stated that good education, manifested in good school grades, in admission to well-known universities like those in Beijing and in graduating from these universities is considered as a step in achieving social security and social advancement and is a common expectation from relatives and friends. It can be understood as a very important "cultural capital" in Bourdieu's sense, which is thought of as hopefully paying off in the future and allowing the accumulation of "economic capital".

---

153 A very recent, though surprisingly short paper by Gan et al. (2012) shows that "more years of education is a risk factor for recurrent major depressive disorders in Chinese women" (991).

154 Lei Feng (雷锋 / 雷鋒) (probably 1940-1962) was a soldier of the People's Liberation Army. Unkown until his death, he became a national hero in the nationwide, posthumous propaganda campaign "Learn from Comrade Lei Feng", initiated in 1963. He was portrayed as a socialist model citizen, characterized as selfless, modest and devoted to Mao Zedong and his ideas. It is disputed whether a soldier named Lei Feng ever existed, but at least it has to be assumed that the 'model citizen' with the specific characteristics is a construction (For further reading on Lei Feng see for example Chen 1965, Reed 1995, Edwards 2010).

Education as a Specific Form of 'Capital'

Pierre Bourdieu broadened the classical Marxian theory of capital by subdividing it into four dimensions. These dimensions are marked as economic, cultural, social and symbolic:

> These fundamental social powers are, according to my empirical investigations, firstly economic capital, in its various kinds, secondly cultural capital or better, informational capital, again in its different kinds; and thirdly two forms of capital that are very strongly correlated, social capital, which consists of resources based on connections and group membership, and symbolic capital, which is the form the different types of capital take once they are perceived and recognized as legitimate (Bourdieu 1987b: 3-4).

Education is subsumed into the category of cultural capital, while subdivided into three more specific subcategories of "incorporated cultural capital", "institutionalized cultural capital" and objectified cultural capital".[155] The "incorporated cultural capital" regards the accumulation of knowledge both from the family background and through formal education in school and university, which leads to certain forms of incorporation, i.e. it becomes an inseparable part of the individual and cannot be sold, inherited or exchanged with someone else. "Institutionalized cultural capital" on the other hand manifests itself in "title and position", i.e. in school- or university-diplomas, which are objective credentials of cultural capital (Rössel & Beckert-Zieglschmid 2002: 498). A great amount of cultural capital is seen as something special and distinguished, because it can be converted into other forms of capital, namely in social capital and the even more important economical capital which promises social and economical profit (Bourdieu 2000: 221). A basic condition for this conversion into other forms of capital is a comparatively complex, market-based society within the paradigm of capitalism (Calhoun 1993:68); a condition which is doubtlessly fulfilled in modern, urban China. Crossley (2001) defines cultural capital as "not such a flexible or transferable currency as money", but nevertheless it can be "cashed in for employment, which then pays off in money (Crossley 2001: 97).

Bourdieu explains that the acquisition of education in order to increase cultural capital needs both time and a specific form of "socially constituted libi-

---

155 This third category, "objectified cultural capital", which manifests itself in the acquisition of items like books, musical instruments or art, is not in the main focus of my interest for this analysis.

do, a *libido sciendi*" (ibid. 219; italics in original). This *libido sciendi*, according to Bourdieu, potentially demands all forms of hardship and sacrifices. In the Chinese context and in accordance with my data, I suggest that these hardships emerge in the form of stress and pressure, thus leading to depression. For example, university students are always in a situation of pressure, for the next exam will surely come soon, a condition caused by what Woronov calls a "harrowing testing system" (Woronov 2008: 417). Simultaneously they feel the pressure from their families because, as an only child, all the hopes and dreams not only for their individual, but also concerns the future and the status (or 'face') of the whole family is projected on them. Furthermore, they constantly compete with their peers for the highest amount of accumulated cultural capital, both incorporated and institutionalized.

But university students are not the only demographic that feel this kind of pressure. Graduates now working are also subjected to pressure and stress. The liberalization of the economy made it necessary to compete with others for the best positions in the best companies. For the early 1990s, Lin and Lai describe that only 1.6% of the urban work force was in the private sector (Lin & Lai 1995: 1134), leaving a large majority employed in governmental 'work units' (*danwei* 单位). These work units restricted competition for professional careers while offering life-time employment, housing, food, energy fuel, health care, leisure activities, schooling and job opportunities for the worker's children, substantial retirement pension, and so forth (ibid. 1133). In today's Beijing, one can suppose that these *danwei* are an exception and a relict of the past. Consequently, the competition for occupation and career is in a full swing. Education is a requirement, and additionally, it is regarded as capital which has to be profitably invested in a steep professional career. This professional career and its benefits further allow the individual to acquire symbolic capital enabling them to compete with its social group. This symbolical capital in modern Beijing mostly consists of apartments, private cars and expensive electronic devices.[156] These items were common topics in young Beijinger's conversation; they were discussed as being very expensive, yet as very essential 'must-haves'.

---

156 To enumerate the three big items (san dajian 三大件) is a Chinese concept to refer to the three most desirable products. As Yan (2000) explains, during the 1960s and 1970s these three items were wristwatches, bicycles and sewing machinese, while in the 1980s colour television, refrigerators and washing machines were most desired. For the 1990s he identified telephones, air conditioners and VCRs as the three big items.

Stress and Depression as Downside of the Chinese Education System

As already pointed out, the Chinese education system is mainly focused on elite-selection. Several recently published articles discuss the Chinese educational system and its crucial role for social mobility (for example Dello-Iacovo 2009, Wang & Morgan 2009, Maurer-Fazio 2006, Lin and Zhang 2006). It is commonly characterized as emphasising memorization, regularly carrying out exams and thus putting pressure on pupils and students. Nevertheless, among my informants I also witnessed the notion that pressure is understood as something indispensable for learners, a view which was reflected, for example, by a 29 year old female postgraduate student:

> A certain level of pressure is good for students, because it pushes them to better achievements. This leads to progress. But the level of pressure one can cope with varies individually, so one has to find the appropriate level of pressure, otherwise too much pressure will arise. (Interview with a female postgraduate student; Böke: Fieldwork 2010/2011).

Teachers and parents or other relatives with their high expectations put great pressure on students to succeed in school and university because failure is associated not only with the individual, but with family and even national shame (Davey et al. 2007: 385, 387).

During an expert interview with Doctor Sun, while asking if there is a connection between the prevalence of depression and the level of education, another doctor temporarily sitting with us suddenly intervened, switched from Chinese to English and explained that

> your observation reveals a big problem of the Chinese education system. There is a special character of the Chinese people: when they get something, they are not happy but want to get more. For example in university, the always want to be number one. The Chinese education system supports this competitiveness. That's why people with higher education are not satisfied with their achievements (Interview with a Chinese doctor in Clinic A; Böke: Fieldwork 2010/2011).

Although there is an awareness of the problems of stress and pressure for Chinese students, reforms carried out in the last decade solve these problems only superficially. Despite intending to create a less exam-oriented education system and to enhance diverse and flexible assessment, the reality shows that students still have to carry a heavy academic burden (Lou 2011: 74).

Education has a greater importance aside from achievements in school or university because the professional career depends largely from the success in the education system: education "plays an important signalling role and is also used as screening device" by Chinese employers (Wang & Morgan 2009: 477; also see Meng & Wang 2005: 47). More fundamentally, if children and youth out of rural areas show their ability for higher education, they have a better opportunity to leave the countryside and settle down in a city legally as students are granted urban residency permits (Brown 2006: 762). For all these reasons, the competition for good jobs is difficult and begins early in school and university. However, it is not regarded as a fate but as a situation where the individual is responsible to be active, as a 25 year old graduate informant of Dong Liang (2005) describes:

> Finding a job nowadays, however, is extremely competitive, so I think that young people have to dare to be bold of vision and courageous action, be willing to study and to keep on the look out for what's out there in the market (Dong 2005: 84).

Concluding, one can say that in China, education is widely regarded as a main road to social mobility and stratification and therefore the individual, as well as the whole extended family, are anxious to achieve good accomplishments.

Gender-specific Peculiarities: 'Superior Births' and 'Superior Mothers'

Chinese medicine developed a special sub-discipline dedicated to women's issues, the so called *fuke* (妇科). As Charlotte Furth (1999) reveals, this sub-discipline, at least for a very long time of Chinese history,

> reveals itself as a social practice not dominated by the role of the elite doctor, [but] where the management of illness might also appear as a domestic skill, as amateur literati learning, as a humble craft or as a religious practice based on ritual (ibid. 3).

According to her, *fuke* never was at the centre of medical culture in imperial China, and the management of gestation and birth remained at least partially outside the circle of male medical specialists (ibid. 301-303).

For today's urban China, the statistical data and the informal interviews reveal that women partially use different medical systems than men, especially with regard to gynaecology and paediatrics. Women stated frequently that they namely trust Western medicine instead of Chinese medicine in "women's issues". My female research assistant was able to collect further information; with her, the participants more openly revealed that for gynaecological issues, they generally prefer Western examination methods and for pregnancy and childbirth, they prefer Western hospitals. One has to keep in mind that official health politics do not encourage home-birth (Mander 2010: 570) and in some provinces, as in the Zhejiang province, home-births are even prohibited (Qiu et al. 2010: 2). This is true for urban areas or zones with a comparatively high degree of centralization; however, in remote areas, at least a few years ago, home-births could still be seen as the standard, although there has been an increase in hospital births, too (Harris et al. 2007: 118). However, I like to emphasize that there is another important reason for women's preference for Western medicine in gynaecology and childbirth aside from the legal status. I argue that the perception of reproduction and childbirth is deeply influenced by societal discourses concerning 'quality'.[157]

"Superior Births" and "Superior Mothers" as Strategies for Raising Population Quality

On the 16th September 2011, the British newspaper 'The Telegraph' published an article by its journalist Malcolm Moore announcing that "China dramatically reduces death in Childbirth".[158] Doctor Luo from a hospital in the city of Yiwu, located in south-eastern China, was quoted with the following statement:

---

157 For a brief overview about the concept of 'quality' in reproductive medicine I refer to Wahlberg 2008.
158 Online version of 'The Telegraph'; http://www.telegraph.co.uk/news/worldnews/asia/china/8768481/ China-dramatically-reduces-death-in-childbirth.html ; last access 20.06.2012.

"One of the reasons for the improvement is regular pregnancy checks. [...] We check on the foetus eight times before birth and we have been constantly updating our medical equipment. We have also improved our care for newborns, and can now look after premature babies who weigh as little as 4lbs, which would have been unthinkable a decade ago." Dr Luo said [...] that "only a few narrow-minded women" would prefer a home delivery.[159]

Beside the doubtlessly great achievement of raising the survival rate of newborns, this quote illustrates the discourse on pregnancy and childbirth, encouraging women to trust in modern, scientific methods and institutions and equating other opinions and preferences with narrow-mindedness.

As Lisa Handwerker (2002: 310) puts it, the One-Child-Policy in China ironically intensified the cultural stigmatization of barren couples and increased the pressure to have at least the one permitted child. Ayo Wahlberg (2010: 378-380) adds that a child not only increases the 'quality' of life of the former childless couple, but that also the "superior birth", "superior childrearing" and "superior education" of that child increases the quality of life of the whole society which, as Wahlberg points out, puts parents and especially women under pressure in order to meet these requirements. Additionally, couples are subjected to societal and 'governmental' control and supervision. This 'self-governing' in order to create a 'superior individual' for a 'superior society' is another manifestation of the specific mode of power which Foucault called 'governmentality' (Foucault 2003: 820-821; also see chapter 7).

The demand for 'high quality offspring' is combined with the promotion of scientific, Western techniques in prenatal examinations, during childbirth and in baby care (Handwerker 2002: 307-308);

In clinical settings, pregnant women, who are considered primarily responsible for giving birth and raising a superior single child, are exposed to educational materials promoting a morally and physically superior baby. [...] Materials range from practical discussion of prenatal care, including nutrition, to more complex concerns about genetics and heredity (ibid. 308).

Additionally, there is not only a discourse on superior children, but also a discourse on "superior women" or "superior mothers". Guo (2010) describes exemplarily, how the Chinese state launched the campaigns 'China's 10 Outstanding Mothers' (Zhongguo shida jiechu muqin 中国十大杰出母亲) and "under-

---

159 ibid.

takes creative action to resynchronize social roles and values" (ibid. 47). These outstanding mothers have to meet certain criteria; aside from party loyalty and patriotism, they have to be modern, open for innovations and new development as well as supporters of scientific methods (ibid. 49).

For Beijing, as already pointed out, there is a massive presence of Western gynaecological clinics and birth and childcare facilities. Advertisement is omnipresent, for example billboards in subway-stations (see Fig. 32). Furthermore, at least in the *Haidian* District[160] where I conducted a relevant part of my observation and where I lived during my stays in Beijing, one could easily find several modern medical institutions and clinics for maternal and child care (Fig. 34). These institutions were obviously highly frequented because long queues of people in front of the reception desk and crowded parking lots could be observed.

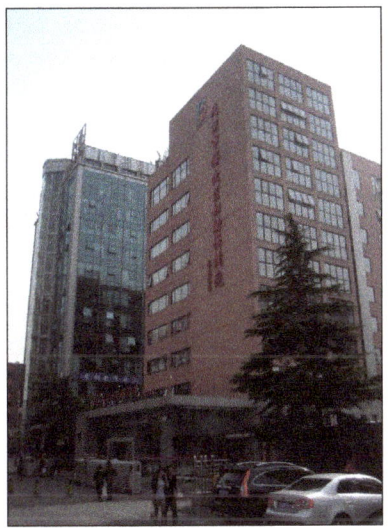

Fig. 34: The "Haidian District healthcare clinic for mothers and infants" *(haidianqu fuyou boajian yuan* 海淀区妇幼保健院*) (Böke: Fieldwork 2010/2011).*

---

160 However, I am sure that this is not a special feature of this city district. Every other district in a big Chinese city with a comparable social composition of young, middle-class couples should host similar institutions.

Consequently, it can be estimated that women in an urban environment both feel a pressure from 'outside' and a desire from 'inside' to meet the expectations. As the 'quality' of the single child, according to political and societal discourse, is best ensured in institutions applying scientific technologies (for example Western clinics), it is consequent to observe a deeper trust in these institutions than in Chinese medical institutions. And as the requirements for women and mothers do imply a preference for scientific and modern technology, equalling other opinions with backwardness and narrow-mindedness, Chinese urban women logically utilize Western medical institution for gynaecology and childbirth.

Summarizing, one can state that there are specific factors creating pressure and stress which are inherent to men and women while some factors affect both sexes.

A couple, in addition to their own child, potentially has to support both sets of in-laws; due to the One-Child-Policy there are no siblings who can share this burden and it puts both men and women under pressure. The same is true for the more general perception of an accelerated lifestyle, leading to collisions between ideas of individual freedom and personal happiness on one hand, and societal realities, political restrictions and familial claims on the other. Educational success and the accumulation of cultural capital also are consumptive for both sexes, and to a certain extent, this is also true for career and occupational expectations. However, men are especially subjected to this kind of pressure, because on the one hand, the role model of the husband as the main breadwinner of the family is still active, and on the other hand, women are limited in their careers through a "glass ceiling" which keeps them out of top positions (Fong 2002: 1102). Fong explains that women not only have to face a "glass ceiling", but are also situated upon a "glass floor", which protects them from social decline (ibid).[161] Men are neither stopped by glass ceilings, nor supported by glass floors. Accordingly, competition, pressure and stress, in order to increase or keep the social status, are merely a problem of men in modern urban China. While women are eager to marry 'upward' on the social ladder, men in contrast (especially those out of remote areas or with only minor symbolic, cultural or economic capital) have the more principal problem of finding a suitable bride.

---

161 She explains that women "enjoy the protection of a glass floor created by the hypergamous marriage system, by gender norms that favour non-elite women in the educational system, and by the rapidly expanding market for feminine jobs in the service and light industry sectors. This glass floor makes it less likely that women will sink to the bottom of society, into poverty, crime, and unemployment (Fong 2002: 1102).

Women on the other hand have to meet certain ideals of beauty in order to marry upward. They are required to be "beautiful, healthy, gentle, chaste, and youthful" (Xia & Zhou 2003: 237). As mothers, they are additionally challenged by ideas of 'superior births' and 'superior mothers', putting them under pressure in order to meet these societal and familial expectations.

8. Conclusion: Chinese Medicine Between Change and Persistence

> "Chinese Medicine is deeply rooted in our culture. It is our cultural heritage."
> (Dr. Zhang, Clinic A)
>
> "There is no true Chinese Medicine anymore; it is too much influenced by modernity."
> (77 year old interviewee in Haidian District)

Chinese Medicine and the idea of emotions as pathogenic agents both have their roots in ancient Chinese philosophy. However, in modern urban China, these ideas are subjected to change and adjustment.

Regarding the human emotions, the two most influential classical philosophies in China, Confucianism and Daoism, both aim in the same direction: namely to avoid emotional excess in order to maintain and preserve life. However, as demonstrated in the analysis of selected philosophical treatises in chapter one, these schools of thoughts approach this issue very differently. Confucianism wants people to live according to moral principles (for example filial piety and benevolence) and thereby take action. Emotional excess is to be actively avoided by acting according to ritual, law and moral code. It only permits a specific amount of emotionality in accordance with specific situations. Emotional instability is regarded as a personal weakness and the preservation of emotional equilibrium is seen as an individual's responsibility. Not only does the individual profit from emotional equilibrium but the whole society depends on harmonious individuals and families, as these institutions are the foundation of the whole society. Daoism on the contrary, demands 'acting through non-acting' (*wu wei* 無為) as a recipe for a long life. Involvement with the world, and thus emotional experience, is regarded as harmful for the human body; accordingly, a natural primordial condition should be achieved. Emotional expression is regarded as infringing upon the Daoist demand for being 'true' or 'genuine' (*zhen* 真), a state which is believed to finally lead to immortality.

This twofold condemnation of emotional utterance represented in these influential Chinese schools of thoughts, founded roughly 3000 years ago, still has an impact on the perception of emotionality in modern urban China. However, history and societal change have had further influences, so that the perception of emotions in urban China fluctuates between change and persistence.

The concluding remarks encompass three parts. First, I summarize my main findings regarding the common perception of Chinese medicine among Beijing inhabitants. Second, I give a short overview on my informant's perception of the pathogenic quality of emotions and the causal relationship between emotionality and illness and briefly compare these attitudes to the statements on emotions and illness expressed in Chinese philosophy and medical theory. Finally, I indicate and discuss three group-specific peculiarities as an outcome of my data analysis: namely, age-specific peculiarities in the perception of depression as emotion-related illness; second, education-specific peculiarities in the notion of stress, pressure and depression; and thirdly, gender-specific peculiarities in the use of Chinese and Western medical institutions.

Common Perception of Chinese Medicine in Beijing

For the people of the Chinese capital, Chinese medicine is one option among others: Aside from Chinese medicine and Western medicine, they stated that many other medical institutions, for example Tibetan, Mongolian or Miao medicine, are available in Beijing.[162] To the question about the utilization of medical help in the last year, 12% answered that they solely used Chinese medicine, 13% used both Chinese and Western medicine. So one quarter of the survey participants used Chinese medicine during the last year, compared to 33% using Western medicine (the remaining 42% have not seen a doctor in the last year). Chinese medicine is thought of as having specific qualities. The most often mentioned quality looks like a disadvantage at first glance: Chinese medicine is regarded as slow, whereas Western medicine is regarded as fast. However, this 'slowness' of Chinese medicine is connected with ideas of being more thorough, focusing more on the roots or causes of the illness (whereas Western medicine is thought of as focusing solely on symptoms), and being without side-effects. Consequently, this slowness is regarded as the main advantage of Chinese

---

162 Interestingly, no other 'foreign' medical system like Ayurveda or others was mentioned.

medicine in opposition to Western medicine. Looking at the Likert-Scales measuring attitudes on Chinese medicine (Chapter 6), one finds that the perception of Chinese medicine in the sample is normally distributed, with the majority being undecided yet probably satisfied with Chinese medicine, and only a small amount of outliers either rejecting it completely or praising Chinese medicine exuberantly.

Regarding the knowledge of Chinese medical concepts one notices striking differences between the different concepts. Whereas three quarters did not know the disease category of the 'Six Evils', 40% did not know the concept of the 'Five Phases' and only a minority of approximately 20% did not know the concept of the 'Seven Emotions'. Obviously, educational background is an important variable in this context. The higher the educational qualification, the better was the knowledge of Chinese medical concepts. The main source of knowledge was, according to the self-reports, television infotainment shows regarding Chinese medicine. These television shows were perceived critically by medical experts of Chinese medicine. While conceding that these shows spread medical knowledge and arouse publicity, the experts stated that these shows are dangerous because of the superficiality and their empty promises of simple solutions. These medical experts regarded themselves as important sources of medical knowledge, emphasizing public lessons and lectures. However, medical experts were only regarded as one source among others by the survey participants.

Educational backgrounds and economical situations not only were a relevant factor for the self-reported knowledge of medical concepts, but also for the self-reported utilization of Chinese medicine. Contrary to the common perception of indigenous medicines as medicine for the poorer, economically marginalised parts of society, at least in Beijing this is not detectable. The higher the income, the higher the probability that survey participants visited Chinese medical institutions, whereas the lower the income, the more people utilized Western medicine. Medical experts explained that this may be due to a certain 'image' of Chinese medicine, which created hype among middle-class white-collar-workers and among well-educated younger urban inhabitants.

The familiarity with the concept of the 'Seven Emotions' – the best-known concept among survey participants – indicates that emotions are commonly regarded as issues in connection with health.

Common Perception of the Connection Between Emotions and Illness

I outlined in chapter two that emotions were regarded as potentially influencing the balance of the body in ancient Chinese philosophical texts of different philosophical schools. Ancient medical texts from different centuries, ranging from the most important texts like the *Huangdi neijing* or *Nanjing* to less popular texts like the *Piwei lun*, already more specifically regard emotions as influencing the bodily circulation of *qi* and blood, causing disharmony and potentially leading to illness. Modern medical textbooks outline distinct connections between specific organs and individual emotions, postulating pathologic working mechanisms. However, this seems not only to be book-wisdom or expert-knowledge; during the survey, people strongly affirmed questions about the pathologic potential of emotions. I collected a broad variety of emotions perceived as potentially pathogenic and recorded different statements about the danger of being overly emotional. Anger, mainly manifested in the two terms *nu* (怒) and *shengqi* (生气), was regarded as especially dangerous and potentially pathogenic. Other emotions like pressure and stress were perceived as problems for members of specific social groups.

In accordance with many survey participants, some medical experts estimated emotions as the main cause for illnesses in general, others emphasized that specific social groups are especially in danger of falling ill due to emotional instability. In urban Chinese society, there is a broad consensus about the perception of emotions as potentially causing illnesses. Additionally, there is also agreement on the most dangerous emotion (anger) and on the organs most likely to be influenced and injured by emotions. Classical medical texts, modern textbooks and common people's statements all emphasize that, although theoretically all organs can be influenced, the heart and the liver are especially vulnerable to emotional upheaval.

Group-specific Peculiarities

The group-specific peculiarities are of special interest. I differentiate between age-specific, education-specific and gender-specific peculiarities. The perception of Chinese medicine in general is age-specific; younger Chinese urban inhabitants seem to be more interested in Chinese medicine than older people. Additionally, the perception of depression as an emotion related illness is completely different among different age cohorts. Stress and pressure are widely regarded as issues for well-educated younger inhabitants, thereby additionally forming an education-specific issue. The utilization of Chinese and Western medicine clearly has a gender-dimension which namely manifests in women's utilization of Western medicine, specifically in the domains of gynaecology and baby care.

Most of the informants stated the impression that younger generations are the main supporters of Chinese medicine in an urban environment like Beijing. These generations were also more open towards my questions and medical experts emphasized the popularity of Chinese medicine among younger people and their interest in indigenous medical beliefs. Older people by contrast were characterized by medical experts as well as by lay people as more reluctant and skeptical as they experienced periods in Chinese history where 'traditional' and 'cultural' were abandoned, namely the Great Leap Forward and the Cultural Revolution. The socialisation under 'specific historical conditions' is also, according to my interpretation, the reason for the different estimation of depression. Whereas older generations generally avoided this topic and did not regard depression as an illness related to emotions, this was the most common issue among younger survey participants (20-29 years). Older generations experienced a different mode of power, where depression was coined not as an illness, but as a crime directly aimed at the absolute ruler and therefore punishable. Younger generations obviously did not experience these historic episodes albeit they face a mode of power more set on governing instead of ruling. The new aim is not to create submissive subjects of a ruler or a sovereign, but to create self-governing subjects, who feel a duty to exhaust their individual capacities, preserve their health and thereby not only improve their individual quality, but also the quality of the whole society.

This notion of quality is strongly connected with the second group-specific observation. The improvement of individual and societal quality puts great pressure and stress on young, well-educated urban individuals. Beside demands by the family network, for example the support for old parents which due to the One-Child-Policy means a great burden for couples, there is also the impression of education as a very important form of investment; an idea which makes education a cultural capital. Families invest heavily in the education of children, hoping that one day this investment in cultural capital pays off in good jobs and successful professional careers and thus manifest itself in economic capital. This puts the individual under great pressure to meet familial and societal expectations and to win in the competition for the admission to the best universities, for the best grades, and for the most prestigious and best-paid jobs.

A third dimension is gender-related. Women use Western medicine more often than men, because they prefer Western medicine for gynaecological issues and childbirth. They do so because of pressure from 'outside' and desire from 'inside'. The One-Child-Policy increases the hopes and expectations for that single child; hence, women are eager to give the best starting position by choosing Western medical institutions which are strongly promoted by the government. The state strongly supports the position that Western scientific and modern institutions are best for 'superior births' of 'superior children' (see chapter 7). Additionally, the construction of 'ideal women' and 'ideal mothers' functions as role model, which many Chinese urban women want to embrace. The idea of 'superior births' and 'superior children' to enhance the quality of the society and simultaneously the rejection of different opinions as 'backward' and 'narrow-minded' permits no free choice for many women. Consequently, Western medical institutions are the first choice in issues related to gynaecology and childbirth.

Outlook

The pressure and stress felt by the well-educated young urban inhabitants, doubtlessly a very important social group for the economic development of every society, is also in Chinese popular media increasingly discussed. For example, on the homepage of a Hong Kong-based television broadcaster, stress and work-related pressure are accused as especially dangerous to male life-quality[163], and on a homepage hosted by the Chinese Google equivalent *baidu*百度, one finds a "Top ten of China's most stressful cities" (*quanguo yali zui da de shi da chengshi*全国压力最大的十大城市)[164]. Additionally, the author of the internet blog "Chinese Dream" identifies pressure and depression as the curse of a whole generation and writes fatalistically on May 25th 2011:

> For Chinese people now it is become extremely common to cross the whole country several times a year. No leisure time; only business going on and going on fast. I remember Shanghai's Friday night talking at the bar: 'You heard this story? The thirty-year-old living on the corner? He died recently, left wife and kids behind. Died out of stress.'

---

163 http://news.ifeng.com/society/2/detail_2010_10/24/2881369_0.shtml ; last access 20.12.2011
164 http://wenku.baidu.com/view/c375a107eff9aef8941e0646.html ; last access 20.12.2011.

> This is an awesomely awesome life I have indeed. People dying out of stress, selling their soul and brothers for a ride on the other side, getting massage – or whatever it means – every night, getting hungry only to get fed again, buying and spending and fucking around. Tell me people, what is the meaning of a Chinese life again?[165]

Hence, by looking at these public discourses, one can estimate the present importance of this topic for the broader public. Additionally, there is a demand for further ethnological research, as these issues will deeply influence the future of Chinese society.

In modern urban China, one can assess an interesting mixture of persistence in specific Chinese medical thought and changes in the perception of illnesses and in the utilization of Chinese and Western medicine.

My analysis shows that certain aspects of Chinese medicine are, one might say, still prevalent among a modern, cosmopolitan urban society like the one in Beijing. The identification of emotions as potentially pathogenic, especially in connection with a perception of balanced emotionality as the best way to avoid the pathogenic impact of emotions, is an idea which not only dates back several thousand years, but which is also regarded as important in modern Beijing. Anger is regarded as the most dangerous emotion among my informants; and liver and heart are assessed as the most endangered organs by the urban inhabitants, in total accordance with ancient and recent texts on Chinese medicine.

Older generations, for political reasons, are characterized as reluctant towards Chinese medicine. However, among younger generations, Chinese medicine is becoming more and more popular; the younger, well-educated generations utilise Chinese medicine to cure ailments related to 'urban lifestyle' such as stress, pressure and depression, which are no longer stigmatized due to cultural and political implications. Chinese medicine is widely regarded as, and has to envision itself, between the two poles of persistence and change.

---

165   http://chinesedream.over-blog.com ; last accessed 20.12.2011.

9. Appendices

Appendix 1:

The questionnaire used in the survey

尊敬的先生/女士，您好！我正在为一个博士研究项目进行调查，此项调查是关于中医，以及在中医体系内疾病与情绪的联系。所有问题的答案无对错之分，希望您能根据自己的实际情况如实地填写。而且问卷调查结果将仅只用于研究，我将严格遵守有关法规，对您的个人信息予以保密。真诚感谢您的合作与帮助！

01. 您知道情志吗? → □ 知道 / □ 不知道

    01a. 您都知道什么情志 (情绪)?

1 _____ 2 _____ 3 _____ 4 _____ 5 _____ 6 _____ 7 _____ 其他 _____

02. 情志出问题会引发疾病吗? → □ 会 / □ 不会

    02a. 您认为哪些疾病是情志导致的?

1 _____ 2 _____ 3 _____ 4 _____ 其他 _____

03. 情志(情绪)会影响脏腑吗? → □ 会 / □ 不会

    03a. 您认为什么情绪会对应影响如下脏腑?

情志 _____ → 脏腑：肝	情志 _____ → 脏腑：胃
情志 _____ → 脏腑：心	情志 _____ → 脏腑：膀胱
情志 _____ → 脏腑：脾	情志 _____ → 脏腑：小肠
情志 _____ → 脏腑：肺	情志 _____ → 脏腑：大肠
情志 _____ → 脏腑：肾	情志 _____ → 脏腑：三焦
情志 _____ → 脏腑：胆	其他 _____

04. 您知道《黄帝内经》吗? → □ 知道 / □ 我听说过，但是具体不清楚 / □ 不知道

      04a. 您觉得这本书重要吗?
→ □ 重要 → 为什么?_____
→ □ 不重要 → 为什么?_____

05. 您知道"五行学说"吗?
→ □ 知道 / □ 我听说过，但是具体不清楚 / □ 不知道

      05a. "五行学说"是什么意思?
      → _____

06. 您知道"六邪"吗?
→ □ 知道 / □ 我听说过，但是具体不清楚 / □ 不知道

      06a. "六邪"是什么?
      → _____

07. 您知道"七情"吗?
→ □ 知道 / □ 我听说过，但是具体不清楚 / □ 不知道

      07a. "七情"是什么?
      → _____

08. 北京有哪些医学体系?
□ 中医 □ 藏医 □ 蒙医 □ 苗医 □ 西医 □ 其他 _____

      08a. 去年您曾使用过以上哪种医学体系治病?
      → _____
      为什么采用这种医学体系?_____

09. 您知道"精神疗法"吗?
→ □ 知道 / □ 我听说过，但是具体不清楚 / □ 不知道

    09a. 您觉得"精神疗法"是什么意思?
→ _____

10.您从哪种途径获得过中医方面的知识?
□电视　□报纸　□书籍　□亲友告知　□医生　□网络　其他 _____

您是否赞成以下论断!　　(1我完全不赞成 **2** 我不赞成 **3** 我不确定
　　　　　　　　　　　　4 我赞成 **5**我完全赞成)

题目	1	2	3	4	5
11. 身体出问题会引发疾病.	1□	2□	3□	4□	5□
12. 内部器官出问题会引发疾病.	1□	2□	3□	4□	5□
13. 中医比西医更好.	1□	2□	3□	4□	5□
14. 情志影响健康.	1□	2□	3□	4□	5□
15. 情志出问题可以引发疾病.	1□	2□	3□	4□	5□
16.中医对情志引发的疾病疗效比西医好.	1□	2□	3□	4□	5□
17. 情志影响疾病.	1□	2□	3□	4□	5□
18. 六邪是导致疾病的重要原因.	1□	2□	3□	4□	5□
19. 七情是导致疾病的重要原因.	1□	2□	3□	4□	5□
20. 人们可以控制情志.	1□	2□	3□	4□	5□
21. 西医比中医更科学.	1□	2□	3□	4□	5□
22. 西医比中医更现代.	1□	2□	3□	4□	5□
23. 情志不会损害健康.	1□	2□	3□	4□	5□
24.不节制的情志对身体很危险.	1□	2□	3□	4□	5□
25. 如果一个人出现情志的问题他应该去看精神治疗医师.	1□	2□	3□	4□	5□
26. 如果一个人出现情志的问题他应该去看神经科的医生.	1□	2□	3□	4□	5□
27. 情志会损害脏腑.	1□	2□	3□	4□	5□

性别：□男　　□女　　　年龄：_____　　　　　民族：_____

您从事什么职业_____
您的最高学历_____

您的月收入是: □1000 元以下　□1000-2000元　□2000-3000元　□3000-4000元
　　　　　　　□4000-5000元　□5000元 以上　　　　　　谢谢您!

Appendix 2:

Social statistics of the survey participants:

Sum total of survey participants: 253

Age cohorts:

20-29: 85 individuals
30-39: 44 individuals
40-49: 51 individuals
50-59: 46 individuals
60-69: 13 individuals
70+: 14 individuals
>> age cohort 60+ : 27 individuals

Educational background:

University graduates: 85 individuals
Higher middle school graduates: 118 individuals
Lower middle school graduates (end of compulsory education): 21 individuals
Primary school education: 14 individuals
No statement: 15 individuals

Income class:

Less than 1000 Yuan RMB per month: 21 individuals
1000-2000 Yuan RMB per month: 75 individuals
2000-3000 Yuan RMB per month: 80 individuals
3000-4000 Yuan RMB per month: 30 individuals
4000-5000 Yuan RMB per month: 12 individuals
More than 5000 Yuan RMB per month: 25 individuals
no statement: 10 individuals

Appendix 3:

Information on medical experts and medical institutions

Dr. Zhang, 48, ♂
Dr. Wen, 31, ♀
Dr. Sun, 37, ♂
Dr. Liu, 28, ♂
Dr. Wang, 24, ♂ } Clinic A
Dr. Li, 30, ♂
Dr. Song, 25, ♂
3 staff members,
between 25 and 59, all ♀

Dr. Zhou, 50, ♀
Dr. Hong, 51, ♂ } Clinic B
Clinic manager, 43, ♂

Dr. Feng, 30, ♀
Dr. Ding, 39, ♀ } Clinic C
Dr. Liang, 44, ♂

Student 1 (postgraduate), ♀, 27
Student 2, ♀, 20
Student 3, ♀, 22 } Students of the Beijing University
Student 4, ♂, 21   of Chinese Medicine
                      (北京中医药大学)

The names of the doctors, according to their own request, are all pseudonyms.

Description of Clinic A:
A small size clinic mainly treating disorders which would be biomedically denoted as stress-related or psychosomatic. Practitioners here mainly use acupunc-

ture, moxibustion and meditation techniques. This clinic was focusing on a middle class clientele and was located in the Haidian district.

Description of Clinic B:
This Clinic is a mid-size clinic, open to a broader public, where different "well known doctors" had their weekly consultation hours and which was supplied with a pharmacy selling herbal drugs prepared according to Chinese medical theory.

Description of Clinic C:
This hospital is one of the main treatment and research institutions of Chinese medicine in Beijing. Up to 8000 patients a day, according to their own statistics, visit this hospital. This hospital invests up to 10 million euro p.a. for psychological research (according to own description).

10. References

AKAHORI AKIRA (1989): The Interpretation of Classical Chinese Medical Texts in Contemporary Japan: Achievements, Approaches, and Problems. In: UNSCHULD, PAUL U. (ed.): *Approaches to Traditional Chinese Medical Literature*. Dordrecht: Kluwer, 19-27.

ANDERSON, E.N. (1990): *The Food of China*. New Haven: Yale University Press.

ANDREWS, BRIDIE (1994): Tailoring Tradition: The Impact of Modern Medicine on Traditional Chinese Medicine, 1887-1937. In: ALLETON, VIVIANE & ALEXEÏ VOLKOV (ed.): *Notions et perceptions du changement en Chine*. (Mémoires de l'institute des hautes etudes Chinoises, Volume XXXVI), Paris: De Boccard, 149-166.

APPADURAI, ARJUN (1990): Topographies of the Self: Praise and Emotion in Hindu India. In: LUTZ, CATHERINE A. & LILA ABU-LUGHOD (Eds.): *Language and the Politics of Emotions*. Cambridge: Cambridge University Press, 92-112.

BARNES, LINDA (2007*)*: *Needles, herbs, gods, and ghosts. China, healing, and the West to 1848*. Cambridge: Harvard University Press.

BARNES, PATRICIA M., BLOOM, BARBARA & RICHARD L. NAHIN (2008): Complementary and Alternative Medicine Use Among Adults and Children: United States 2007. *National Health Statistics Report* 12 (National Centre for Health Statistics).

BARRY, CHRISTINE A. (2005): Pluralism of Provision, Use and Ideology. In: JOHANNESSEN, HELLE (ed): *Multiple medical realities*. New York: 89-104.

BAUER, WOLFGANG (1971): *China und die Hoffnung auf Glück. Paradiese, Utopien, Idealvorstellungen*. München: Carl Hanser Verlag.

BEDFORD, ERROL (1986): Emotions and Statements about them. In: HARRÉ, ROM (Hrsg.): *The Social Construction of Emotion*. Oxford: Basil Blackwell, 15-31.

BENEDICT, RUTH. (1934): *Patterns of Culture*. Boston.

BERKOWITZ, LEONARD & EDDIE HARMON-JONES (2004): Toward an Understanding to the Determinants of Anger. *Emotion* 4(2): 107-130.

BÖKE, MARTIN (2008): *Die Rolle der Emotionen im traditionellen chinesischen Medizinsystem*. (Kölner Ethnologische Beiträge Bd. 27), Köln.

BOND, M. H. (1993): Emotions and their Expression in Chinese Culture, *Journal of Nonverbal Behaviour*, 17 (4), S. 245-262.

--- (1987) (Hrsg.): *The Psychology of the Chinese People*, New York.

BOURDIEU, PIERRE (2010): Distinctions. A Social Critique of the Judgement of Taste. (Translated by Richard Nice). London & New York: Routledge.

---- (2000): Ökonomisches, kulturelles und soziales Kapital. In: BAUMGART, FRANZJÖRG (ed.): *Theorien der Sozialisation*. Bad Heilbrunn: Klinkhardt. 217-231.
---- (1987a): *Die feinen Unterschiede. Kritik einer gesellschaftlichen Urteilskraft*. Frankfurt a.M.: Suhrkamp.
---- (1987b): What makes a social class? On the theoretical and practical existence of groups. *Berkeley Journal of Sociology* 32: 1-18.
---- (1979): *La distinction. Critique sociale du jugement*. Paris: Editions de Minuit.
BROWN, PHILIP H. (2006): Parental Education and Investment in Children's Human Capital in Rural China. *Economic Development and Cultural Change* 54(4): 759-789.
BURKITT, IAN. (1999): *Bodies of Thought. Embodiment, Identity and Modernity*. London: Sage.
CALHOUN, CRAIG (1993): Habitus, Field, and Capital: The Question of Historical Specificity. In: CALHOUN, CRAIF, LIPUMA, EDWARD & MOISHE POSTONE (eds.): *Bourdieu: Critical Perspectives*. Cambridge: Polity Press. 61-88.
CASIMIR, MICHAEL J. (2009a): On the Origin and Evolution of Affective Capacities in Lower Vertebrates. In: RÖTTGER-RÖSSLER, BIRGIT & HANS J. MARKOWITSCH (eds.): *Emotions as Bio-cultural Processes*. New York: Springer, 55-94.
---- (2009b): "Honor and Dishonor" and the Quest for Emotional Equivalents. In: RÖTTGER-RÖSSLER, BIRGIT & HANS J. MARKOWITSCH (eds.): *Emotions as Bio-cultural Processes*. New York: Springer, 281-316.
CHAN, ADRIAN (2009): *Orientalism in Sinology*. Palo Alto: Academia Press.
CHAN, ANITA (1985): *Children of Mao. Personality Development and Political Activism in the Red Guard Generation*. London: Macmillan.
CHANG, DORIS F., TONG HUIQI, SHI QIJIA, ZENG QIFENG (2005): Letting a Hundred Flowers Bloom: Counseling and Psychotherapy in the People's Republic of China. *Journal of Mental Health Counseling* 27 (2): 104-115.
CHAO, YÜAN-LING (2009): *Medicine and Society in Late Imperial China*. New York: Peter Lang.
CHATURVEDI, S. K., DESAI, GEETHA & DEEPIKA SHALIGRAM (2006): Somatoform Disorders, Somatization and Abnormal Illness Behaviour. *International Review of Psychiatry* 18 (1): 75-80.
CHEN, G.S. (1968): *Lei Feng: Chairman Mao's good fighter*. Beijing: Beijing Foreign Languages Press.
CHEN RUOLING, WEI LI, HU ZHI, QIN XIA, COPELAND, JOHN R. & HARRY HEMMINGWAY (2005): Depression in Older People in Rural China. *Archives of Internal Medicine* 165: 2019-2025.

CHEN XIAOMEI (1994): *Occidentalism: Theory of counter-discourse in post Mao China*. Oxford: Oxford University Press.
CHENG CHUNG-YING (2001): Morality of Daode and Overcoming of Melancholy in Classical Chinese Philosophy. In: KUBIN, WOLFGANG (ed.): *Symbols of Anguish: In Search of Melancholia in China*. (Schweizer Asiatische Studien Vol. 38), Bern: Peter Lang, 77-104.
CHENG, CHUNG-YING & NICOLAS BUNNIN (2002) (ed.): *Contemporary Chinese Philosophy*. Oxford: Blackwell.
CHINA DAILY 09.08.2008: *The Philosophy of Harmony*. (URL: http://www.Chinadaily.com.cn/Olympics/20008-08/09/content_6920168.htm ; last access 31.05.2011).
CONNERTON, PAUL (1989): *How Societies Remember*. Cambrigdge: University Press.
CRONBACH, LEE J. (1951): Coefficient Alpha and the Internal Structure of Tests. *Psychometrika* 16 (3): 297-334.
CROSSLEY, NICK (2001): *The Social Body. Habit, Identity and Desire*. London: Sage.
CROZIER, RALPH C. (1965): Traditional Medicine in Communist China. Science, Communism and Cultural Nationalism. *The China Quarterly* 23: 1-27.
CSORDAS, THOMAS (1990): Embodiment as a Paradigm for Anthropology. *Ethos* 18(1): 5-47.
---- (1994): Introduction. The Body as Representation and Being in the World. In: CSORDAS, THOMAS (ed.): *Embodiment and Experience. The Existential Ground of Culture and Self*. Cambridge: Cambridge University Press, 1-26.
DAMASIO, ANTONIO R. (1994): *Descartes' Error. Emotion, Reason, and the Human Brain*. New York: Avon Books.
DAVEY, GARETH, LIAN, CHUAN DE & LOUISE HIGGINS (2007): The University Entrance Examination System in China. *Journal of Further and Higher Education* 31(4): 385-396.
DE KLOET, JEROEN: (2002): Rock in a Hard Place. In: HEMELRYK DONALD, STEPHANIE, MICHAEL KEANE & YIN HONG (ed.): *Media in China. Consumption, Content and Crisis*. London: RoutledgeCurzon, 93-104.
DELLO-IACOVO, BELINDA (2009): Curriculum and 'Quality Education' in China: an Overview. *International Journal of Educational Development* 29:241-249.
DELURY, JOHN (2008): "Harmonious" In China. *Policy Review* 148: 35-44.
DIEKMANN, ANDREAS (2009): *Empirische Sozialforschung. Grundlagen, Methoden, Anwendungen*. Reinbek: Rowohlt Taschenbuchverlag.
DIRLIK, ARIF (1996a): Chinese History and the Question of Orientalism. *History and Theory* 35 (4): 96-118.

DIRLIK, ARIF (1996b): Ironies, Hegemonies: Notes on the Contemporary Historiography of Modern China. *Modern China* 22 (3): 243-284.
DONG LIANG (2005): "If You Are Ready to Work and Ready to Study, The You'll Find a Job You Like. *Chinese Education and Society* 38(4): 82-84.
DOUGLAS, MARY (1970): *Natural Symbols: Explorations in Cosmology.* Harmondsworth: Penguin Books.
EBENSTEIN, AVRAHAM (2010): The "Missing Girls" of China and the Unintended Consequences of the One Child Policy. *Journal of Human Resources* 45(1): 87-115.
EDWARDS, LOUISE (2010): Military Celebrity in China: The Evolution of 'Heroic and Model Servicemen'. In: EDWARDS, LOUISE & ELAINE JEFFREYS (eds.): *Celebrity in China.* Hong Kong: Hong Kong University Press. 21-44.
EHRENBERG, ALAIN (1998): *La Fatigue d'être soi. Dépression et société.* Paris: Editions Odile Jacob.
---- (2010): *Weariness of the Self: Diagnosing the History of Depression in the Contemporary Age.* Québec: McGill-Queen's Press.
EKMAN, PAUL (1972): Universals and Cultural Differences in Facial Expressions of Emotions. In: COLE, JAMES K. (ed.): *Nebraske Symposium on Motivation 1972.* Lincoln: University of Nebraska Press, 207-285.
---- (1981): Universale emotionale Gesichtsausdrücke. In: KAHLE, GERD (ed.): *Logik des Herzens. Die soziale Dimension der Gefühle.* Frankfurt a.M.: Suhrkamp, 177-186.
---- (1984): Expression and the Nature of Emotion. In: SCHERER, KLAUS R. & PAUL EKMAN (ed.): *Aprroaches to Emotion.* Hillsdale NJ: Lawrence Erlbaum, 319-343.
EKMAN, PAUL & WALLACE FRIESEN (1969): The Repertoire of Nonverbal Behavior: Categories, Origins, Usage, and Coding. *Semiotica* 1(1): 48-98.
---- (1971): Constants across Cultures in the Face and Emotion. *Journal of Personality and Social Psychology* 17(2): 124-129.
EKMAN, PAUL, SORENSON, RICHARD E. & WALLACE FRIESEN (1969): Pan-Cultural Elements in Facial Displays of Emotions. *Science* 164: 86-88.
ENGELFRIET, PETER M. (2000): Linked Faiths, Divergent Paths? Some Remarks on Taoism and Medicine in Late Ming and Early Qing China. In: DE MEYER, JAN A. M. & PETER M. ENGELFRIET (eds.): *Linked Faiths. Essays on Chinese Religions and Traditional Culture in Honour of Kristofer Schipper.* Leiden: Brill, 248-268.
ENGELHARDT, UTE (2000): Longevity Techniques and Chinese Medicine. In: KOHN, LIVIA (ed.): *Daoism Handbook.* Leiden: Brill.
ESCOBAR, JAVIER I., GOMEZ, J. & V. B. TUASON (1983): Depressive Phenomenology in North and South American Patients. *American Journal of Psychiatry* 140: 47-51.

FABREGA, HORACIO (1975): The Need for an Ethnomedical Science. *Science* 189 (4207): 969-975.
---- (1990a): A Plea for a Broader Ethnomedicine. *Culture, Medicine and Psychiatry* 14, 129-132.
---- (1990b): The Concept of Somatization as a Cultural and Historical Product of Western Medicine. *Psychosomatic Medicine* 52: 653-672.
---- (1991): Somatization in Cultural and Historical Perspective. In: KIRMAYER, LAURENCE J. & JAMES M. ROBBINS (eds.): *Current Concepts of Somatization: Research and Clinical Perspective*. (Progress in Psychiatry 31) Washington: American Psychiatric Press, 181-200.
FARQUHAR, JUDITH (1994a): *The Clinical Encouter of Chinese Medicine*. Boulder & Oxford: Westview Press.
---- (1994b): Eating Chinese Medicine. *Cultural Anthropology* 9(4): 471-497
---- (2002): *Appetites. Food and Sex in Post-Socialist China*. Durham: Duke University Press.
FELDMAN, ALLEN (1991): *Formations of Violence. The Narrative of the Body and Political Terror in Northern Ireland*. Chicago: University of Chicago Press.
FLICK, UWE (2010): *Qualitative Sozialforschung. Eine Einführung*. Reinbek: Rowohlt Taschenbuchverlag.
FONG, VANESSA (2002): China's One-Child-Policy and the Empowerment of Urban Daughters. *American Anthropologist* 104(4): 1098-1109.
---- (2004): Filial Nationalism among Chinese Teenagers with Global Identities. *American Ethnologist* 31(4): 631-648.
---- (2007): Parent-Child Communication Problems and the Perceived Inadequacy of Chinese Only Children. *Ethos* 35(1):85-127.
FOUCAULT, MICHEL (2011) [1975]: *Surveiller et punir. Naissance de la prison*. Paris: Gallimard.
---- (2007): *Security, Territory, Population: Lectures at the Collège de France 1977-1978*. New York: Palgrave.
---- (2005): Schriften in vier Bänden. Dits et Ecrits. Band IV 1980-1988. (Herausgegeben von Daniel Defert und François Ewald unter Mitarbeit von Jacques Lagrange). Frankfurt a. M.: Suhrkamp.
---- (2003): Schriften in vier Bänden Dits et Ecrits. Band III 1976-1979. (Herausgegeben von Daniel Defert und François Ewald unter Mitarbeit von Jacques Lagrange). Frankfurt a. M.: Suhrkamp.
---- (1994a): Dits et écrits. III 1976-1979 (Édition établie sous la direction de Daniel Defert et François Ewald). Paris: Edition Gallimard.
---- (1994b): Dits et écrits. IV 1980-1988 (Édition établie sous la direction de Daniel Defert et François Ewald avec la collaboration de Jacques Lagrange). Paris: Edition Gallimard.

Fox, Patricia, Coughlan, Barbara, Butler, Michelle & Cecily Kelleher (2010): Complementary alternative medicine (CAM) use in Ireland: A secondary analysis of SLAN data. *Complementary Therapies in Medicine* 18 (2): 95-103.

Fu Lianzhang (1955): Why our Western-trained doctors should learn Traditional Chinese Medicine. *Chinese Medical Journal* 73 (5), 363-367.

Fung Yu-lan (1983): *A History of Chinese Philosophy*. (Translated by Derk Bodde). Princeton: Princeton University Press.

Furth, Charlotte (1999): A *Flourishing Yin. Gender in China's Medical History, 960-1665.* Berkeley, Los Angeles & London: University of California Press.

Gan Zhaoyun, Li Yihan, Xie Dong, Shao Chunhong, Yang Fuzhong, Shen Yuan, Zhang Ning, Zhang Guanghua, Tian Tian, Yin Aihua, Chen Ce, Lie Jun, Tang Chunling, Zhang Zhuoqiu, Liu Jia, Sang Wenhua, Wang Xumei, Liu Tiebang, Wei Qinling, Xu Yong, Sun Ling, Wang Sisi, Li Chang, Hu Chunmei, Cui Yanping, Liu Ying, Li Ying, Zhao Xiaochuan, Zhang Lan, Sun Lixin, Chen Yunchun, Zhang Yueying, Ning Yuping, Shi Shenxun, Chen Yiping, Kendler, Kenneth S., Flint, Jonathan & Zhang Jinbei (2012): The Impact of Educational Status on the Clinical Features of Major Depressive Disorder Among Chinese Women. *Journal of Affective Disorders* 136: 988-992.

George, Darren & Paul Mallery (2002[4]): *SPSS for Windows Step by Step: A Simple Guide and Reference*. Boston: Allyn & Bacon.

Goldberg, D. P. & K. Bridges (1988): Somatic Presentations of Psychiatric Illness in Primary Care Setting. *Journal of Psychosomatic Research* 32: 137-144.

Graham, A. C. (1990): *Studies in Chinese Philosophy and Philosophical Literature*. (Suny Series in Chinese Philosophy and Culture) Albany: State University of New York Press.

Greenhalgh, Susan (1993): Controlling Births and Bodies in Village China. *American Ethnologist* 21(1): 1-30.

---- (2001): Under the Medical Gaze. Facts and Fictions of Chronicle Pain. Berkeley: University of California Press.

---- (2008): *Just one Child. Science and Policy in Deng's China*. Berkeley: University of California Press.

---- (2011): Governing Chinese Life. From Sovereignty to Biopolitical Governance. In: Zhang, Everett, Kleinman, Arthur & Tu Weiming (eds.): *Governance of Life in Chinese Moral Experience. The Quest for an Adequate Life*. London & New York: Routledge. 146-162.

Guo Yingjie (2010): China's Celebrity Mothers: Female Virtues, Patriotism and Social Harmonie. In: : Edwards, Louise & Elaine Jeffreys (eds.): *Celebrity in China*. Hong Kong: Hong Kong University Press. 45-66.

HAGEN, KURTIS (2003): Xunzi and the Nature of Confucian Ritual. *Journal of the American Academy of Religion* 71 (2), 371-403.
HAMDI, E. AMIN, Y. & M. T. SALEH (1997): Perfomance of the Hamilton Depression Rating Scale in Depressed Patients in the United Arab Emirates. *Acta Psychiatrica Scandinavica* 96 (6): 416-423.
HANDWERKER, LISA (2002): The Politics of Making Modern Babies in China. Reproductive Technologies and the "New" Eugenics. In: INHORN, MARCIA C. & FRANK VAN BALEN (eds.): *Infertility Around the Globe. New Thinking on Childlessness, Gender, and Reproductive Technologies*. Berkeley & Los Angeles: University of California Press. 298-314.
HANSEN, CHAD (1995): Qing (Emotions) 情 in Pre-Buddhist Chinese Thought. In: MARKS, JOEL & ROGER T. AMES (eds.): *Emotions in Asian Thought. A Dialogue in Comparative Philosophy*. Albany: State University of New York, 181-212.
HANSEN, METTE H. (2008): In the Footsteps of the Communist Party: Dilemmas and Strategies. In: HEIMER, MARIA & STIG THØGERSEN (eds.): *Doing Fieldwork in China*. Honolulu: University of Hawai Press, 81-95.
HANSON, MARTA (1997): *Inventing a Tradition in Chinese Medicine: From Universal Canon to Local Medical Knowledge in South China, The Seventeenth to the Nineteenth Century*. (Ph.D. Dissertation, University of Pennsylvania).
---- (1998): Robust Northerners and Delicate Southerners: The Nineteenth-Century Invention of a Southern Wenbing Tradition. *Positions: East Asia Cultures Critique* 6.3: 515-549.
HARPER, DONALD J. (1998): *Early Chinese medical literature: the Mawangdui medical manuscripts*. (The Sir Henry Wellcome Asian Series), London & New York: Kegan Paul International.
HARRIS, AMANDA, YU GAO, BARCLAY, LESLIE, BELTON, SUZANNE, ZWENG WEIYUE, HAO MIN, XU AUQUN, LIAO HUA & ZHOU YUN (2007): Consequences of Birth Policies and Practices in Post-Reform China. *Reproductive Health Matters* 15(30): 114-124.
HENDRISCHKE, BARBARA (2001): Joy and Sadness in Daoism. In: KUBIN, WOLFGANG (ed.): *Symbols of Anguish: In Search of Melancholia in China*. (Schweizer Asiatische Studien Vol. 38). Bern: Peter Lang, 105-141.
HILL, JOHN E. (2009): *Through the Jade Gate to Rome: A Study of the Silk Routes during the Later Han Dynasty, 1st to 2nd Centuries CE*. Charleston: BookSurge.
HINRICHS, T.J. (1998): New Geographies of Chinese medicine. *Osiris* 13: 287-325.
HO, PENG YOKE & F. PETER LISOWSKI (1993): *Concepts of Chinese Science and Traditional Healing Art*. Singapore u.a.
HOBSBAWM, ERIC (1983): Introduction: Inventing Traditions. In: HOBSBAWM,

ERIC & TERENCE RANGER (ed.): *The Invention of Tradition*. Cambridge: Cambridge University Press, 1-14.
HOBSBAWM, ERIC & TERENCE RANGER (1983) (ed.): *The Invention of Tradition*. Cambridge: Cambridge University Press.
HSIEH, ANDREW C. K. & JONATHAN D. SPENCE (1980): Suicide and the family in pre-modern Chinese Society. In: KLEINMAN, ARTHUR & LIN TSUNG-YIN (eds.): *Normal and Abnormal Behaviour in Chinese Culture*. Dordrecht: Reidel Publishing Company, 29-48.
HSU, ELISABETH. (1999): *The Transmission of Chinese Medicine*, Cambridge: Cambridge University Press.
---- (2003): Die drei Körper – oder sind es vier? Medizinethnologische Perspektiven auf den Körper. In: LUX, THOMAS. (ed.): *Kulturelle Dimensionen der Medizin. Ethnomedizin – Medizinethnologie – Medical Anthropology*. Berlin: Reimer, 177-189.
---- (2005): Tactility and the Body in Early Chinese Medicine. *Science in Context* 18(1), 7–34.
---- (2007): The Experience of Wind in Early Medieval Chinese Medicine. *Journal of the Royal Anthropological Institute* 13 (1): 117-134.
---- (2008): The History of Chinese Medicine in the People's Republic of China and its Globalization. *East Asia Science, Technology and Society* 2: 465-484.
HUGHES, NEIL C. (2002): *China's Economic Challenges. Smashing the Iron Rice Bowl*. Armonk: M.E. Sharpe.
HUNT, KATHERINE J., H. F. COELHO, B. WIDER, R. PERRY, S. K. HUNG, R. TERRY & E. ERNST (2010): Complementary and Alternative Medicine Use in England: Results from a National Survey. *International Journal of Clinical Practice* 64 (11): 1496-1502.
IKELS, CHARLOTTE (2004) (ed.): *Filial Piety. Practice and Discourse in Contemporary East Asia*. Stanford: Stanford University Press.
IVANHOE, PHILIP J. & BRYAN W. VAN NORDEN (2001) (ed.): *Readings in Classical Chinese Philosophy*. Cambridge: Hackett Publishing Company.
IZARD, CARROLL E. (1971): *The Face of Emotion*. New York: Appleton-Century-Crofts.
--- (1977): *Human Emotions*. New York: Plenum.
JANKOWIAK, WILLIAM, MOORE, ROBERT & TIANSHU PAN (2012): Institutionalizing an Extended Youth Phase in Chinese Society. Social Class and Sex Differences in the Pursuit of the Personal and the Pragmatic. In: AMIT, VERED & NOEL DYCK (eds.): *Young Men in Uncertain Times*. New York & Oxford: Berghahn, 79-107.
JEWELL, J.A. (1990): Theoretical Basis of Chinese Traditional Medicine. In: HILLIER, S. M.& J. A. JEWELL (ed.), *Health Care and Traditional Chinese Medicine in China, 1800-1982*. London: 221-241.

JI, CHENG YE & CHENG TSUNG (2008): Epidemic increase in overweight and obesity in Chinese children from 1985-2005. *International Journal of Cardiology* 132: 1–10
KAPTCHUK, TED J. (2000): *Chinese Medicine. The Web That Has No Weaver*. London: Rider.
KAWANISHI, YUKIO (1992): Somatization of Asians: An Artifact of Western Medicalization? *Transcultural Psychiatric Research Reviews* 29: 5-36.
KING, BRIAN (1989): *The Conceptual Structure of Emotional Experience in Chinese*. (Unpublished Dissertation Ohio State University).
KIRMAYER, LAURENCE J. & ALLAN YOUNG (1998): Culture and Somatization: Clinical, Epidemiological, and Ethnographic Perspectives. *Psychosomatic Medicine* 60: 420-430.
KLEINMAN, ARTHUR (1978a): What Kind of Model for the Anthropology of Medical Systems? *American Anthropologist* (80) 3: 661-665.
---- (1978b): Concepts and a Model for the Comparison of Medical Systems as Cultural Systems. *Social Science & Medicine* 12: 85-95.
---- (1979): *Patients and Healers in the Context of Culture: An Exploration of theBorderland Between Anthropology, Medicine and Psychiatry*. Berkeley: University of California Press.
---- (1982): Neurasthenia and Depression: A Study of Somatization and Culture in China. *Culture, Medicine and Psychiatry* 6: 117-190.
---- (1986): *Social Origins of Distress and Disease: Depression, Neurasthenia, and Pain in Modern China*. New Haven: Yale University Press.
KLEINMAN, ARTHUR & JOAN KLEINMAN (1994): How Bodies Remember: Social Memory and Bodily Experience of Criticism, Resistance, and Delegitimation Following China's Cultural Revolution. *New Literary History* 25(3): 707-723.
---- (1999): The Transformation of Everyday Social Experience: What a Mental and Social Health Perspective Reveals about Chinese Communities under Global and Local Change. *Culture, Medicine and Psychiatry* 23(1):7-24.
---- (2007): Somatization: The Interconnections in Chinese Society among Culture, Depressive Experience, and the Meanings of Pain. In: LOCK, MARGARET & JUDITH FARQUHAR (eds.): *Beyond the Body Proper. Reading the Anthropology of Material Life*. Durham & London: Duke University Press, 468-474.
KLEINMAN, A. & T. Y. LIN (1980): *Normal and Abnormal Behavior in Chinese Culture*. Dordrecht.
KOVACS, JÜRGEN & PAUL U. UNSCHULD (1998): *Essential subtleties on the silver sea: The Yin-hai jing-wei: a Chinese classic on ophthalmology*. Berkeley: University of California Press.

KÖVECSES, ZOLTÁN (1998): Are there any emotion-specific metaphors? In: ANGELIKI ATHANASIADOU & ELZBIETA TABAKOWSKA (eds.): *Speaking of Emotions: Conceptualization and Expression.* 127-151. Berlin: Mouton de Gruyter.

---- (1995): Metaphors and Folk Understanding of Anger. In: . JAMES A. RUSSEL, JOSÉ-MIGUEL FERNÁNDEZ-DOLS, ANTONY S.R. MANSTEAD & J.C. WELLENKAMP (eds.): *Everyday conceptions of emotions: an introduction to the psychology, anthropology and linguistics of emotion.* 49-71. London: Kluwer.

LAI, GINA (1995): Work and Family Roles and Psychological Well-Being in Urban China. *Journal of Health and Social Behaviour* 36:11-37.

LAM, WILLY (2005): China's 11th five-year plan. A roadmap for China's "harmonious society?" *Association for Asian Research Articles.* (Internet Resource; URL: http://www.asianresearch.org/articles/ 2756.html ; last access 13.06.2012).

LANG, OLGA (1946): *Chinese Family and Society.* New Haven: Yale University Press.

LASH, SCOTT (1991): Genealogy and the Body: Foucault/Deleuze/Nietsche. In: FEATHERSTONE, MIKE, HEPWORTH, MIKE & BRYAN S. TURNER (eds.): *The Body. Social Process and Cultural Theory.* London: Sage. 256-280.

LEDOUX, JOSEPH E. (1995): Emotions: Clues from the Brain. *Annual Review of Psychology* 46: 209-235.

---- (1996): *The Emotional Brain.* New York: Simon and Schuster.

LEE, SING & ARTHUR KLEINMAN (2007): Are Somatoform Disorders Changing with Time? The Case of Neurasthenia in China. *Psychosomatic Medicine* 69: 846-849.

LESLIE, CHARLES. (1976) (ed.): *Asian Medical Systems. A Comparative Study*, Berkeley: University of California Press.

LIKERT, RENSIS (1931): A Technique for the Measurement of Attitudes. *Archives of Psychology* 139: 44-53.

LIN JING & YU ZHANG (2006): Educational Expansion and Shortages in Secondary Schools in China: The Bottle Neck Syndrome. *Journal of Contemporary China* 15(47):255-274.

LIN, KEH-MING & FREDA CHEUNG (1999): Mental Health Issues for Asian Americans. *Psychiatric Services* 50 (6): 774-780.

LIN, KEH-MING, KLEINMAN, ARTHUR, & LIN TSUNG-YI (1980): Overview of Mental Disorders in Chinese Cultures: Reviews of Epidemiological and Clinical Studies. In: KLEINMAN, ARTHUR & LIN TSUNG-YIN (eds.): *Normal and Abnormal Behaviour in Chinese Culture.* Dordrecht: Reidel Publishing Company, 237-272.

LIN NAN & LAI GINA (1995): Urban Stress in China. *Social Science and Medicine* 41(8): 1131-1145.

LIU HAN-PING, LIANG BO, ZHANG HE-MIN, LIU XIAO-YAN & LIU SONG-YAO (2012): Specificity of Auricular Acupoints in Reflecting Changes of Qi and Blood Measured Diffuse Reflectance Spectroscopy. *Journal of Chinese Integrative Medicine* 10(2): 186-192.

LIU, JEELOO (2006): *An Introduction to Chinese Philosophy. From Ancient Philosophy to Chinese Buddhism.* Oxford: Blackwell.

LIU JIAN-MENG, YE RONGWEI, LI SONG, REN AIGUO, LI ZHIWEN, LIU YINGHUI & LI ZHU (2007): Prevalence of Overweight/Obesity in Chinese Children. *Archives of Medical Research* 38: 882-886.

LIU QINGPING (2011): Emotionales in Confucianism and Daoism: A New Interpretation. *Journal of Chinese Philosophy* 38 (1): 118-133.

LIU YANCHI, LIU ZHANWEN 刘燕池, 刘占文 (1998) (ed.): *Zhongyi jichu lilun* 中医基础理论 (Basic Theory of Traditional Chinese Medicine). Beijing: Xueyuan chubanshe.

LOCK, MARGARET. (2007): Medical Anthropology: Intimations fort he Future, in: SAILLENT, F. & S. GENEST (ed.): *Medical Anthropology. Regional Perspectives and Shared Concerns*, Malden, 267-288.

LOU JINGJING (2011): Suzhi, Relevance and the New Curriculum. A Case Study of One Rural Middle School in Northwest China. *Chinese Education and Society* 44(6): 73-86.

LU JIN, RUAN YE, HUANG YUEQIN, YAO JIAN, DANG WEIMIN & GAO CHANGQING (2008): Major Depression in Kunming: Prevalence, Correlates and Co-Morbidity in a South-Western City of China. *Journal of Affective Disorders* 111: 221-226.

LU XING (2004): *Rhetoric of the Chinese Cultural Revolution. The Impact on Chinese Thought, Culture and Communication.* Columbia: University of South Carolina Press.

LUKES, STEVEN (2005): *Power. A Radical View.* New York: Palgrave.

LUPHER, MARK (1995): Revolutionary Little Red Devils: The Social Psychology of Rebel Youth 1966-1967. in: ANNE BEHNKE KINNEY (ed.): *Chinese Views of Childhood.* 321-344. Honululu: University of Hawaii Press.

LUPTON, DEBORAH (1998): *The Emotional Self. A Sociocultural Exploration.* London: Sage Publications.

LUTZ, CATHERINE (1986): Emotion, Thought, and Estrangement: Emotions as Cultural Category. *Cultural Anthropology* 1(3): 287-309.

---- (1988): *Unnatural Emotions. Everyday Sentiments on a Micronesian Atoll and their Challenge to Western Theory*. Chicago: University of Chicago Press.

---- (1996): Engendered Emotion. Gender, Power, and the Rhetoric of Emotional Control in American Discourse. In: HARRÉ, ROM & W. GERROD PARROTT (ed.): *The Emotions. Social, Cultural and Biological*

Dimensions. London: Sage Publications, 151-170.
LUTZ, CATHERINE & LILA ABU-LUGHOD (1990) (ed.): *Language and the Politics of Emotion*. Cambridge: Cambridge University Press.
LUTZ, CATHERINE & GEOFFREY M. WHITE (1986): The Anthropology of Emotions. *Annual Review of Emotions* 15: 405-436.
LYON, MARGOT L. (1998): The Limitations of Cultural Constructionism in the Study of Emotion. In: BEDELOW, GILLIAN & SIMON J. WILLIAMS (ed.): *Emotions in Social Life. Critical Themes and Issues*. London & New York: Routledge, 39-59.
MAO ZEDONG (1953): *Mao Zedong xuanji di san juan* 毛澤東選集第三卷 (Selected Works of Mao Zedong Vol. III). Beijing: Renmin chubanshe.
MANDER, ROSEMARY (2010): The Politics of Maternity Care and Maternal Health in China. *Midwifery* 26: 569-572.
MATTEN, MARC ANDRÉ (2009*): Die Grenzen des Chinesischen. National Identitätsstiftung im China des 20. Jahrhunderts*. Wiesbaden: Harrassowitz.
---- (2011): The Worship of General Yue Fei and His Problematic Creation of a National Hero in Twentieth Century China. *Frontiers of History in China* 6(1):74-94.
MAURER-FAZIO, MARGARET (2006): In Books One Finds a House of Gold: education and labor market outcomes in urban China. *Journal of Contemporary China* 15(47): 215-231.
MAUSS, MARCEL. (1935): Les techniques du corps. *Journal de psychologie,* 32, 271-293.
MEAD, MARGARET. (1928): *Coming of Age in Samoa*. New York.
---- (1930): *Growing up in New Guinea: A Comparative Study of Primitive Education*. New York.
---- (1935): *Sex and Temperament in Three Primitive Societies*. New York.
MEES, ULRICH (2006): Zum Forschungsstand der Emotionpsychologie – eine Skizze. In: SCHÜTZEICHEL, RAINER (ed.): *Emotionen und Sozialtheorie. Disziplinäre Ansätze*. Frankfurt a.M. & New York: Campus, 104-123.
MENG DAHU & WANG SHUO (2005): Diploma Screening, Human Capital and Employment of Junior College Graduates: An Analysis based on Research. *Meitan Higher Education* 23(4): 46-49.
MERSKEY, HAROLD & FREDERICK G. SPEAR (1967): *Pain: Psychological and Psychiatric Aspects*. London: Bailliere, Tindall and Cassell.
MERTON, ROBERT K. (1949): *Social Theory and Social Structure*. New York: Free Press.
MERTON, ROBERT K. & ELINOR BARBER (2004): *The Travels and Adventures of Serendipity*. Princeton: Princeton University Press.
MESSNER, ANGELIKA (2006): Emotions, Body, and Bodily Sensation within

an Early Field of Expertise Knowledge in China. In: SANTAGELO, PAOLO (ed.) in Cooperation with Ulrike Middendorf: *From Skin to Heart. Perceptions of Emotions and Bodily Sensations in Traditional Chinese Culture*. Wiesbaden: Harrassowitz, 41-66.

MICHEL, WOLFGANG (1993): Frühe westliche Beobachtungen zur Moxibustion und Akupunktur. *Sudhoffs Archiv* 77, 2: 193-222.

--- (2005): Far Eastern Medicine in Seventeenth and Early Eighteenth Germany. *Studies in Languages and Cultures* 20 (Faculty of Languages and Cultures, Kyushu University): 67-81.

MONSCHEIN, YLVA (1989): Lu Xuns Erzählung *Yao* oder die Wirksamkeit eines Placebos. In: KUBIN, WOLFGANG (ed.): *Aus dem Garten der Wildnis. Studien zu Lu Xun (1881-1936)*. Bonn: Bouvier, 29-46.

NANJING ZHONGYI XUEYUAN 南京中医学院 (Nanjing Academy of Traditional Chinese Medicine) (1958) (ed.): *Zhongyixue gailun* 中医学概论 (Introduction to Chinese Medicine). Beijing: Renmin weisheng chubanshe.

NATIONAL BUREAU OF STATISTICS OF CHINA 中华人民共和国国家统计局 (2011) ChinaStatistical Yearbook 2010 中国统计年鉴 2010 (http://www.stats.gov.cn/tjsj/ndsj/2010/indexch.htm , last accessed at 16.11.2011).

NETTLETON, SARAH & JONATHAN WATSON (1998): The Body in Everyday Life. An Introduction. In: NETTLETON, SARAH & JONATHAN WATSON (ed.): *The Body in Everyday Life*. London & New York: Routledge, 1-23.

NYLAN, MICHAEL (2001): On the Politics of Pleasure. *Asia Major* 14, 73-124.

OCHSNER, KEVIN N. & MATTHEW D. LIEBERMAN (2001): The Emergence of Social Cognitive Neuroscience. *American Psychologist* 56 (9): 717-734.

OCHSNER, KEVIN N. & JAMES J. GROSS (2005): The Cognitive Control of Emotions. *Trends in Cognitive Sciences* 9 (5): 243-247.

OTS, THOMAS (1987): Aneignung durch Umdeutung – Zur Rezeption der traditionellen chinesischen Medizin in Deutschland. *Curare* 10: 169-195.

---- (1990): The angry liver, the anxious heart and the melancholy spleen. The Phenomenology of Perceptions in Chinese Culture. Culture, Medicine and Psychiatry, 14 (2), 21-58.

---- (1994): The silenced body, the expressive Leib: on the dialectic of mind and life in Chinese cathartic healing, in: CSORDAS, THOMAS (ed.): *Embodiment and Experience*. Cambridge, 116-136.

---- (1999): *Medizin und Heilung in China - Annäherungen an die traditionelle chinesische Medizin*. Berlin: Reimer.

PAN, DA'AN (2003): The Tao of a peaceful mind: the representation of emotional health and healing in traditional Chinese literature. *Mental Health, Religion and Culture* 6 (3): 241-259.

PAN, LYNN (1990): *Sons of the Yellow Emperor. The Story of the Overseas*

Chinese. London: Secker & Warburg.

PARK, LAWRENCE & DEVON HINTON (2002): Dizziness and Panic in China. Associated Sensations of Zangfu Organ Disequilibrium. *Culture, Medicine and Psychiatry* 26: 225-257.

PARKER, GORDON, GEMMA GLADSTONE & KUAN TSEE CHEE (2001): Depression in the Planet's Largest Ethnic Group: The Chinese. *American Journal of Psychiatry* 158:857-864.

PEARSON, VERONICA (1995): *Mental Health Care in China. State Policies, Professional Services, and Family Responsibilities.* London: Gaskell

PHILLIPS, MICHAEL R., LIU HUAQING & ZHANG YANPING (1999): Suicide and Social Change in China. *Culture, Medicine and Psychiatry* 23: 25-50.

PHILLIPS, MICHAEL R., ZHANG JINGXUAN, SHI QICHANG, SONG ZHIQIANG, DING ZHIJIE, PANG SHUTAO, LI XIANYUN, ZHANG YALI & WANG ZHIQING (2009): Prevalence, Treatment and Associated Disability of Mental Disorders in Four Provinces in China During 2001-05: An Epidemiological Survey. *The Lancet* 373 (9680):2041-2053.

PILKINGTON, KAREN, KIRKWOOD, GRAHAM, RAMPES, HAGEN, CUMMINGS, MIKE & JANET RICHARDSON (2007): Acupuncture for Anxiety and Anxiety Disorders – a Systematic Literature Review. *Acupunture in Medicine* 25(1-2): 1-10.

PLUTCHIK, ROBERT (1982): A psychoevolutionary theory of emotions. *Social Science Information* 21 (4/5), 529-553.

PORKERT, MANFRED (1973): *Die theoretischen Grundlagen der chinesischen Medizin* Wiesbaden: Franz Steiner Verlag.

---- (1976) The Intellectual and Social Impulses Behind the Evolution of Traditional Chinese Medicine. In: LESLIE, CHARLES. (ed.): *Asian Medical Systems: A Comparative Study.* Berkeley: University of California Press, 63-76.

---- (1986) *Die chinesische Medizin.* Düsseldorf, Wien: Econ Verlag.

POWELL, JASON & IAN COOK (2000): "A Tiger Behind, and Coming up Fast": Governmentality and the Politics of Population Control in China. *Journal of Aging and Identity* 5(2): 79-89.

PRITZKER, SONYA (2003): The Role of Metaphor in Culture, Consciousness, and Medicine: A preliminary inquiry into the metaphors of depression in Chinese and Western medical and common language. *Clinical Acupuncture and Oriental Medicine*, 4(1), 11-28.

QIU LIQIAN, LIN JUN, MA YUANYING, WU WEIWEI, QIU LING, ZHOU AIZHEN, SHI WENJUN, LEE, ANDY & COLIN BINNS (2010): Improving the maternal mortality ratio in Zhejiang Province, China, 1988–2008. *Midwifery* 26: 544-548.

RAMESH, M. & XUN WU (2009): Health policy reforms in China: Lessons from Asia. *Social Science and Medicine* 68: 2256-2262.

RAO, DEEPA, YOUNG, M. & R. RAGURAM (2007): Culture, Somatization, and Psychological Distress: Symptom Presentation in South Indian Patients from a Public Psychiatric Hospital. *Psychopathology* 40: 349-355.
REED, GAY GARLAND (1998): Is Lei Feng Finally Dead? The Search for Values in a Time of Reform and Transition. In: AGELASTO, MICHAEL & BOB ADAMSON (eds.): *Higher Education in Post-Mao China*. Hong Kong: Hong Kong University Press. 359-373.
---- (1995): Moral/Political Education in the People's Republic of China: learning through role models. *Journal of Moral Education* 24(2): 99-111.
ROBINET, ISABELLE (2008): Taiji tu. In: PREGADIO, FABRIZIO (ed.): The Encyclopedia of Taoism. (Volume II), Routledge:London, 934-936.
ROJEK, DEAN G. (2001): Chinese Social Control: From Shaming and Reintegration to "Getting Rich is Glorious". In: LIU JIANHONG, ZHANG LENING & STEVEN F. MESSNER (eds.): *Crime and Social Control in a Changing China*. Westport & London: Greenwood. 96-103.
ROSE, NIKOLAS (2011): Biological Citizenship and its forms. In: ZHANG, EVERETT, KLEINMAN, ARTHUR & TU WEIMING (eds.): *Governance of Life in Chinese Moral Experience. The Quest for an Adequate Life*. London & New York: Routledge. 237-265.
---- (2007): *The Politics of Life Itself: Biomedicine, Power and Subjectivity in the Twenty First Century*. Princeton: Princeton University Press.
ROSE, NIKOLAS & CARLOS NOVAS (2005): 'Biological Citizenship'. In: ONG, AIHWA & STEPHEN J. COLLIER (eds.): *Global Assemblages: Technology, Politics, and Ethics as Anthropological Problems*. Malden: Blackwell Publishing. 439-463.
RÖSSEL, JÖRG & CLAUDIA BECKERT-ZIEGLSCHMID (2002): Die Reproduktion kulturellen Kapitals. *Zeitschrift für Soziologie* 31(6): 497-513.
RÖTTGER-RÖSSLER, BIRGIT (2002): Emotion und Kultur: Einige Grundfragen. *Zeitschrift für Ethnologie* 127, 147-162.
---- (2004): *Die kulturelle Modellierung des Gefühls. Ein Beitrag zur Theorie und Methodik ethnologischer Emotionsforschung anhand indonesischer Fallstudien*. Münster: Lit Verlag.
ROSALDO, MICHELLE (1984): Toward an anthropology of self and feeling. In: SHWEDER, RICHARD A & ROBERT A. LEVINE (ed.): *Culture Theory: Essays on Mind, Self and Emotion*. Cambridge: Cambridge University Press, 137-157.
RYDER, ANDREW G., YANG JIAN, ZHU XIONGZHAO, YAO SHUQIAO, YI JINYAO, HEINE, STEPHEN J. & R. MICHAEL BAGBY (2008): The Cultural Shaping of Depression: Somatic Symptoms in China, Psychological Symptoms in North America? *Journal of Abnormal Psychology* 117 (2): 300-313.
SAID, EDWARD W. (1979): *Orientalim*. New York: Vintage books.
SANTANGELO, PAOLO (1999): Emotions and the Origin of Evil in Neo-

Confucian Thought. In: EIFRING, HALVOR (ed.): *Minds and Mentalities in Traditional Chinese Lierature*. Beijing: Culture and Art Publishing House, 184-316.
---- (2003): Sentimental Education in Chinese History. An Interdisciplinary Textual Research on Ming and Qing Sources. Leiden & Boston: Brill.
---- (2005): Evaluation of Emotions in European and Chinese Traditions: Differences and Analogies. *Monumenta Serica* 53: 401-427.
SCHEID, VOLKER. (2002): *Chinese Medicine in Contemporary China. Plurality and Synthesis*, Durham & London.
---- (2006): Chinese Medicine and the Problem of Tradition. *Asian Medicine* 2 (1): 59-71.
SCHEPER-HUGHES, NANCY (1992*): Death without weeping. The Violence of Everyday Life in Brazil*. Berkeley: University of California Press.
SCHEPER-HUGHES, NANCY & MARGARET LOCK (1987): The Mindful Body: A Prolegomenon to Future Work in Medical Anthropology. *The Journal of the Royal Anthropological Association* 12 (1): 95-118.
SCHÜTZEICHEL, RAINER (2006): Emotionen und Sozialtheorie – eine Einleitung. In: SCHÜTZEICHEL, RAINER (ed.): *Emotionen und Sozialtheorie. Disziplinäre Ansätze*. Frankfurt a.M. & New York: Campus, 7-26.
SCHWARCZ, VERA (1986): *The Chinese enlightenment: intellectuals and the legacy of the May Fourth Movement of 1919*. Berkeley: University of California Press.
SELIGMAN, REBECCA & RYAN A. BROWN (2010): Theory and Method at the Intersection of Anthropology and Cultural Neuroscience. *Social Cognitive and Affective Neuroscience* 5 (2-3): 130-137.
SETHI, B. B. (1986): Epidemiology of Depression in India. *Psychopathology* 19 (Suppl. 2): 26-36.
SHANGHAI ZHONGYIYAO DAXUE 上海中医药大学(Shanghai University of Traditional Chinese Medicine) (2002) (ed.): *Zhongyi neikexue* 中医内科学 (Internal Traditional Chinese Medicine). Shanghai: Shanghai zhongyiyao daxue chubanshe.
SHEN, FRANCES C., WANG, YU-WEI & JANE L. SWANSON (2011): Development and Initial Validation of the Internalization of Asian American Stereotype Scale. *Cultural Diversity and Ethnic Minority Psychology* 17 (3): 283-294.
SINGER, M. & H. BAER (1995): *Critical Medical Anthropology*. New York: Baywood.
SMITH, KIDDER (2003): Sima Tan and the Invention of Daoism, "Legalism", et cetera. The *Journal of Asian Studies* 62 (1): 129-156.
SMITH, W. LYNN (2009): *The Mind-Body Interface in Somatization. When Symptom becomes disease* (with Patrick W. Conway and Jonathan O. Cole). Lanham a.o.: Jason Aronson.

So, Joseph K. (2007): Somatization as Cultural Idiom of Distress: Rethinking Mind and Body in a Multicultural Society. *Counselling Psychotherapy Quarterly* 21 (2): 167-174.
Solomon, Robert C. (1981): Emotionen und Anthropologie: Die Logik emotionaler Weltbilder. In: Kahle, Gerd (ed.): *Logik des Herzens. Die soziale Dimension der Gefühle*. Frankfurt a. M.: Suhrkamp. 233-253.
Spencer, Michael S., Chen, Juan, Gee, Gilbert C., Fabian, Cathryn G. & David T. Takeuchi (2010): Discrimination and Mental Health-Related Service Use in a National Study of Asian Americans. *American Journal of Public Health* 100 (12): 2410-2417.
Spielberg, Petra (2007): Schul- und Komplementärmedizin. Miteinander statt nebeneinander. *Deutsches Ärzteblatt* 104 (46): 3148.
Stein, Nancy L. & Keith Oatley (1992) (ed.): *Basic Emotions*. Hove: Lawrence Erlbaum.
Strickman, Michel (2002): *Chinese Magical Medicine*. (Edited by Bernard Faure). Stanford, Stanford University Press.
Sun Rongjun (2004): Worry About Medical Care, Family Support and Depression of the Elders in Urban China. *Research on Aging* 26(5):559-585.
Svasek, Maruska (2005): Introduction: Emotions in Anthropology. In: Milton, Kay & Maruska Svasek (ed.): *Mixed Emotions. Anthropological Studies of Feeling*. New York: Berg.
Taylor, Kim (2001): A new, scientific, and unified medicine: civil war in China and the new acumoxa, 1945-1949. in: Hsu, Elisabeth (ed.): *Innovation in Chinese Medicine* (Needhan Institute Studies 3). Cambridge: Cambridge University Press, 343-369.
---- (2004): Divergent Interests and Cultivated Misunderstandings: The Influence of the West on Modern Chinese Medicine. *Social History of Medicine* 17 (1): 93-111.
---- (2005): *Chinese Medicine in Early Communist China, 1945-63. A medicine of revolution*. London & New York: RoutledgeCurzon.
Thøgersen, Stig (2008): Beyond Offical Chinese. Language Code and Strategies. In: Heimer, Maria & Stig Thøgersen (eds.): *Doing Fieldwork in China*. Honolulu: University of Hawai Press, 110-128.
Tseng, Wen-Shing & David Y.H. Wu (1985) (eds.): *Chinese Culture and Mental Health*. Orlando: Academic Press.
Tung, May P. M. (1994): Symbolic Meanings of the Body in Chinese Culture and "Somatization". *Culture, Medicine and Psychiatry* 18 (4): 483-492.
Ulich, Dieter & Philipp Mayring (1992): *Psychologie der Emotionen*. Stuttgart: Kohlhammer.
Unschuld, Paul U. (1979): Naturwissenschaft, Medizin und Marxismus im China des 20. Jahrhunderts. *Curare* 2: 125-136.

---- (1985): *Medicine in China. A History of Ideas*. Berkeley: University of California Press.
---- (1986): *Nan-Ching. The Classic of Difficult Issues*. With commentaries by Chinese and Japanese authors from the third through the twentieth century. Berkeley: University of California Press.
---- (1987): Traditional Chinese Medicine: Some Historical and Epistemological Reflections. *Social Science & Medicine* 24 (12): 1023-1029.
---- (1988): *Introductory Readings in Chinese Medicine*. Dordrecht: Kluwer.
---- (1990): *Forgotten Traditions of Ancient Chinese Medicine*. Brookline: Paradigm Publications.
---- (1991): Die theoretischen Grundlagen der chinesischen Medizin vor der Begegnung mit der westlichen Welt. in: KUBIN, WOLFGANG. (ed.): *Neue Mitteilungen des Seminars für Orientalische Sprachen der Universität Bonn*, Bd. 1, Bonn.
---- (1995): *Huichun. Rückkehr in den Frühling. Chinesische Heilkunde in historischen Objekten und Bildern*. München, New York: Prestel.
---- (2003): *Was ist Medizin?* München: C. H. Beck.
---- (2006): Das Schriftzeichen für *yi*. Zweifacher Anachronismus. *minima sinica* 1: 45-47.
UNSCHULD, PAUL U. & MA KANWEN (1984): Medizinisch-pharmazeutisches Schrifttum. In: CHRISTA HABRICH & JÖRN HENNING WOLF (eds.): *Medizin in China. Katalog zu einer Sonderausstellung im Deutschen Medizinhistorischen Museum Ingolstadt* (Kataloge des Deutschen Medizinhistorischen Museums, Heft 5). Ingolstadt: Albert Stadlmeyer KG: 7-9.
ÜRESIN, YESIM (2008): *Depression und Somatisierung bei türkischen Migrantinnen* (Dissertation University of Hamburg). Hamburg.
WAHLBERG, AYO (2008): Reproductive Medicine and the Concept of 'Quality'. *Clinical Ethics* 3: 189-193
---- (2010): Assessing Vitality: Infertility and Good Life in Urban China. In: YORKE, JON (ed.): *The Right to Life and Value of Life: Orientations in Law, Politics, and Ethics*. Farnham: Ashgate. 371-397.
VANKEEBERGHEN, GRIET (1995): Emotions and the Actions of the Sage: Recommendations for an Orderly Heart in the "Huainanzi". *Philosophy East and West* 45 (4): 527-544.
WANG HUI (2008): *Translating Chinese Classics in a Colonial Context. James Legge and His Two Versions of the Zhongyong* (Worlds of East Asia Welten Ostasiens Mondes de'l Extrème Orient Vol. 13). Bern: Peter Lang.
WANG, NAIXIA & W. JOHN MORGAN (2009) Student Motivation, Quality and Status in Adult Higher Education (AHE) in China. *International Journal of Lifelong Education* 28(4):473-491.

WANG PING (2005): Zur Entstehung des chinesischen Schriftzeichens *wu* 诬 („verleumden") aus dem Zeichen *wu* 巫 („Schamane"). *Orientierungen* 1: 104-108.
WANG SHAOGUANG (2003): Between Destruction and Construction. The First Year of the Cultural Revolution. In: LAW, KAM-YEE (ed.): *The Chinese Cultural Revolution Reconsidered. Beyond Purge and Holocaust.* New York: Palgrave Macmillan. 25-57.
WANG SHU-MING, PELOQUIN, CAROL & ZEEV N. KAIN (2001): Brief Reports: The Use of Auricular Acupuncture to Reduce Preoperative Anxiety. *Anesthesia & Analgesia* 93(5): 1178-1180.
WANG XINYUE 王新月 (2007a) (ed.): *Zhongyi neikexue* 中医内科学 (Internal Traditional Chinese Medicine). Beijing: Gaodeng jiaoyu chubanshe.
---- (2007b) (ed.): *Zhongyi linchuang jichu* 中医临床基础 (Clinical Basics of Traditional Chinese Medicine). Beijing: Gaodeng jiaoyu chubanshe.
WANG ZHIGANG (1991): Taoism and Self-Cultivation. *Journal of Chinese Medicine* 37: 27-30.
WHITE, GEOFFREY M. (1982): The Role of Cultural Explanations in "Somatization" and "Psychologization". *Social Science and Medicine* 16 (16): 1519-1530.
WHYTE, MARTIN KING (1997): The Fate of Filial Obligations in Urban China. *The China Journal* 38: 1-31.
WHYTE, MARTIN KING & WILLIAM L. PARISH (1984): *Urban Life in Contemporary China*. Chicago & London: The University of Chicago Press.
WINKLER, CATHY (1994): Rape Trauma. Contexts of Meaning. In: CSORDAS, THOMAS (ed.): *Embodiment and Experience. The Existential Ground of Culture and Self*. Cambridge: Cambridge University Press, 248-268.
WIERZBICKA, ANNA (1999) *Emotions across Languages and Cultures. Diversity and Universals*. Cambridge and Paris: Cambridge University Press.
WOOLFOLK, ROBERT L. & LESLEY A. ALLEN (2007): *Treating Somatization. A Cognitive-Behavioral Approach*. New York & London: Guilford Press.
WORONOV, T. E. (2008): Raising Quality, Fostering "Creativity": Ideologies and Practices of Education Reform in Beijing. *Anthropology and Education Quarterly* 39(4):401-422.
WU, DAVID Y. H. (1982): Psychotherapy and Emotion in Traditional Chinese Medicine. In: MARSELLA, ANTHONY J. & GEOFFREY M. WHITE (eds.): *Cultural Conceptions of Mental Health and Therapy*. Dordrecht: Reidel Publishing Company, 285-301.
XUE, CHARLIE C., ZHANG, ANTHONY L., LIN, VIVIAN, DA COSTA, CLIFF &

DAVID F. STORY (2007): Complementary and Alternative Medicine Use in Australia: A National Population-Based Survey. *The Journal of Alternative and Complementary Medicine* 13 (6): 643-650.

XIA, YAN R. & ZHI G. ZHOU (2003): The Transition of Courtship, Mate Selection, and Marriage in China. In: HAMON, RAEANN R. & BRON B. INGOLDSBY (eds.): *Mate Selection Across Cultures*. London: Sage. 231-246.

XIANG SHILIN (2008): A study on the theory of "returning to the original" and "recovering nature" in Chinese philosophy. *Frontiers of Philosophy in China* 3 (4): 502-519.

XIE ZHUFAN (2003): *On the Standard Nomenclature of Traditional Chinese Medicine*. Beijing: Foreign Language Press.

XU, JUDY & YUE YANG (2009): Traditional Chinese medicine in the Chinese health care system. *Health Policy* 90: 133-139.

XU WEIWEI, IGOR SHEIMAN, WYNAND VAN DEN VEN & WEI ZHANG (2011): Prospects for regulated competition in the health care system: what can China learn from Russia's experience? *Health Policy and Planning* 26: 199-209

XU XIAOQUN (1997): 'National Essence' vs 'Science': Chinese Native Physicians' Fight for Legitimacy, 1912-37. Modern Asian Studies 31 (4): 847-877.

YAN YUNXIANG (2000): The Politics of Consumerism in Chinese Society. In: WHITE, TYRENE (ed.): *China Briefing, 1998-2000*. Armonk: M.E. Sharpe, 179-193.

---- (2003): *Private Life Under Socialism. Love, Intimacy, and Family Change in a Chinese Village, 1949-1999*. Stanford: Stanford University Press.

---- (2005): The Individual and Transformation of Bridewealth in Rural North China. *Journal of the Royal Anthropological Institute* 11(4):637-657.

---- (2006): Girl Power: The Women and the Waning of Patriarchy in Rural North China. *Ethnology* 45(2): 105-123.

---- (2009): *The Individualization of Chinese Society*. (London School of Economics Monographs on Social Anthropology, Vol. 77). Oxford & New York: Berg.

YANG NIANQUN (2011): Memories of the Barefoot Doctor System (translated by Everett Zhang). In: ZHANG, EVERETT, KLEINMAN, ARTHUR & TU WEIMING (eds.): *Governance of Life in Chinese Moral Experience. The Quest for an Adequate Life*. London & New York: Routledge. 131-145.

YAO XINZHONG (2000): *An Introduction to Confucianism*. Cambridge: Cambridge University Press.

YU NING (1995): Metaphorical Expressions of Anger and Happiness in English and Chinese. *Metaphor and Symbolic Activity* 10(2):59-92.

ZANE, NOLAN & MAY YEH (2002): The Use of Culturally-Based Variables in Assessment: Studies on Loss of Face. In: KURASAKI, KAREN S., OKAZAKI, SUMIE & STANLEY SUE (eds.): *Asian American Mental Health. Assessment Theories and Methods*. New York: Kluwer, 141-158.

ZHAN, HEYING JENNY (2006): Joy and Sorrow: Explaining Chinese Caregiver's Reward and Stress. *Journal of Aging Studies* (20):27-38.

ZHANG DAINIAN & EDMUND RYDEN (2002): *Key Concepts in Chinese Philosophy*.New Haven: Yale University Press.

ZHANG, EVERETT (2011a): Introduction. Governmentality in China. In: ZHANG, EVERETT, KLEINMAN, ARTHUR & TU WEIMING (eds.): *Governance of Life in Chinese Moral Experience. The Quest for an Adequate Life*. London & New York: Routledge. 1-30.

---- (2011b): The Truth about the Death Toll of the Great Leap Famine in Sichuan: An Analysis of Maoist Sovereignty. In: ZHANG, EVERETT, KLEINMAN, ARTHUR & TU WEIMING (eds.): *Governance of Life in Chinese Moral Experience. The Quest for an Adequate Life*. London & New York: Routledge. 62-79.

ZHANG TONG & BARRY SCHWARTZ (2003): Confucius and the Cultural Revolution: A study in Collective Memory. In: OLICK, JEFFREY K. (ed.): *Continuities, Conflicts, and Transformations in National Retrospection*. Durham & London: Duke University Press. 101-127.

ZHANG YANHUA (2007a): *Transforming Emotions with Chinese Medicine*. New York: Suny.

---- (2007b): Negotiating a Path to Efficacy at a Clinic of Traditional Chinese Medicine. *Culture, Medicine and Psychiatry* 31: 73-100.

ZHOU XIAOLU, DERE, JESSICA, ZHU XIONGZHAO, YAO SHUQIAO, CHENTSOVA-DUTTON, YULIA E. & ANDREW G. RYDER (2011): Anxiety Symptom Presentations in Han Chinese and Euro-Canadian Outpatients: Is Distress Always Somatized in China? *Journal of Affective Disorders* 135(1-3): 111-114.

ZÜRCHER, ERIK (2007³): *The Buddhist Conquest of China. The Spread and Adaptation of Buddhism in Early Medieval China*. Leiden: Brill.

References of the Classical Chinese texts cited:

Guanzi 管子
　in: Sturgeon, Donald: Chinese Text Project
　[Internet source http://ctext.org/guanzi ; last access 03.11.2011].
Huainanzi 淮南子
　in: Sturgeon, Donald: Chinese Text Project
　[Internet source http://ctext.org/huainanzi ; last access 03.11.2011].
Huangdi neijing 黃帝內經,
　in: Sturgeon, Donald: Chinese Text Project
　[Internet source http://ctext.org/huangdi-neijing ; last access 03.11.2011].
Liji 禮記
　in: Sturgeon, Donald: Chinese Text Project
　[Internet source http://ctext.org/liji ; last access 03.11.2011].
Lunyu 論語
　in: Sturgeon, Donald: Chinese Text Project
　[Internet source http://ctext.org/analects ; last access 03.11.2011].
Nanjing 難經
　in: Sturgeon, Donald: Chinese Text Project
　[Internet sourcehttp://ctext.org/nan-jing ; last access 03.11.2011].
Piwei lun 脾胃論
　in: Unschuld, Paul (1988): *Introductory Readings in Chinese Medicine*. Dordrecht: Kluwer.
San yin ji yi bingzheng fang lun 三因極一病證方論
　in: Unschuld, Paul (1988): *Introductory Readings in Chinese Medicine*. Dordrecht: Kluwer.
Xunzi 荀子
　in: Sturgeon, Donald: Chinese Text Project
　[Internet source http://ctext.org/xunzi ; last access 03.11.2011].
Yixue yuan liu lun 醫學源流論
　in: Unschuld, Paul (1990): *Forgotten Traditions of Ancient Chinese Medicine*. Brookline: Paradigm Publications.
Zhuangzi 莊子
　in: Sturgeon, Donald: Chinese Text Project
　[Internet source http://ctext.org/zhuangzi ; last access 03.11.2011].
Zhu bing yuan hou lun 諸病源侯論
　in: Unschuld, Paul (1985): *Medicine in China: A History of Ideas*. Berkeley: University of California Press.

www.ingramcontent.com/pod-product-compliance
Ingram Content Group UK Ltd.
Pitfield, Milton Keynes, MK11 3LW, UK
UKHW021827140426
5217IPUK00016B/1239